NOV 1 3 1993

DATE DUE

DEC 8 1993	
JAN 1 3 1994	
FEB 2 8 1994	
MAR 9 1994	
APR 1 1994	
APR 8 1994	
APR 2 2 1994	
MAY 1 6 19	
MAY 1 6 1994	
JUN 6 1994	
JUL 7 1994	
BRODART	Cat. No. 23-221

D0403044

150
MOST-ASKED
QUESTIONS
ABOUT
OSTEOPOROSIS

Also by Ruth S. Jacobowitz

150 Most-Asked Questions About Menopause

Managing Your Menopause
(with Wulf Utian, M.D., Ph.D.)

Daly City Public Library
Daly City, California

DISCARDED

150 Most-Asked Questions About Osteoporosis

WHAT WOMEN
REALLY WANT TO KNOW

Ruth S. Jacobowitz

Hearst Books • New York

W

616.716
JAC

The ideas, suggestions, and answers to questions in this book are not intended to substitute for the help and services of a trained professional. All matters regarding your health require medical consultation and supervision, and following any of the advice and procedures in this book should be done in conjunction with the services of a qualified health professional.

The names and biographical information referred to in anecdotes in this book have been changed to protect the identity of the individuals concerned.

Copyright © 1993 by Ruth S. Jacobowitz

The song lyrics that appear on page 142 are excerpted from "It Isn't Enough" from the musical production *The Roar of the Greasepaint—The Smell of the Crowd*. Words and Music by Leslie Bricusse and Anthony Newley © Copyright 1965 (Renewed) Concord Music Ltd., London, England. TRO—Musical Comedy Productions, Inc., New York, controls all publication rights for the U.S.A. and Canada. Used by permission.

All rights reserved. No part of this book may be reproduced or utilized in any form or by any means, electronic or mechanical, including photocopying, recording, or by any information storage or retrieval system, without permission in writing from the Publisher. Inquiries should be addressed to Permissions Department, William Morrow and Company, Inc., 1350 Avenue of the Americas, New York, N.Y. 10019.

It is the policy of William Morrow and Company, Inc., and its imprints and affiliates, recognizing the importance of preserving what has been written, to print the books we publish on acid-free paper, and we exert our best efforts to that end.

Library of Congress Cataloging-in-Publication Data

Jacobowitz, Ruth S.
   150 most-asked questions about osteoporosis : what women really
want to know / Ruth S. Jacobowitz.—1st ed.
     p.   cm.
   Includes bibliographical references and index.
   ISBN 0-688-12334-1 (acid-free paper)
   1. Osteoporosis—Miscellanea.   I. Title.   II. Title: One hundred
fifty most-asked questions about osteoporosis.   III. Title: One
hundred and fifty most-asked questions about osteoporosis.
RC931.O73J33   1993
616.7'16—dc20

93-15426
CIP

Printed in the United States of America
First Edition

1 2 3 4 5 6 7 8 9 10

Foreword

June 18, 1990, represents the defining moment in the women's health movement. On that day, the General Accounting Office, an investigative arm of the U.S. Congress, reported on the status of research on women at the National Institutes of Health. The report found that not only were women underrepresented in most clinical trials, but also that the diseases that affect women were not part of the national research agenda. Clearly, women's health issues have not been receiving the medical research funding and attention they deserve.

These findings reverberated throughout the women's community and sparked the women's health movement. The women's health movement, an unofficial coalition of organizations, policymakers, grassroots leaders, and health care experts, gave birth to a series of legislative initiatives and national policies that focus attention on women's health issues.

Foreword

A women's health issue has been defined as a health problem, condition, or disease that is unique to women; is more prevalent in women; is more serious among women; and has risk factors and interventions that are different for women.

By these criteria, osteoporosis stands as a foremost women's health problem. From a medical, physiological, psychological, sociological, and economic perspective, osteoporosis affects women differently than men. Women's bones are generally lighter and less dense than men's, and women experience menopause, which drastically influences their bone health. Osteoporosis leads to physical changes, such as severe curvature of the spine and loss of height, which affect a woman's body image and, often, her self-esteem. Because of generally lower income and lack of health care reimbursement for necessary testing, women encounter significant barriers to early diagnosis. And because women have a longer life expectancy, the likelihood of developing fractures associated with osteoporosis is greatly increased.

Since osteoporosis primarily affects women, it is easy to understand why this disease has been largely ignored.

Osteoporosis is a bone-thinning disease in which the skeleton becomes so fragile that the slightest movement, even a cough or sneeze, can cause a bone to fracture. Osteoporosis affects more than 25 million Americans, 80 percent of whom are women. Because osteoporosis is a "silent disease" that can progress undetected for decades, often the first sign of the disease is a fracture. Each year, this disease leads to 1.5 million bone fractures, typically of the hip, spine, and wrist, although any bone can be affected.

The characteristically stooped posture often evident in older women and men is the result of osteoporotic fractures of the vertebrae, the bones that make up the spine. Vertebral fractures cause the spine to collapse and curve unnaturally. The majority of hip fractures are also the result of osteoporosis and can lead to the disease's most serious consequences— loss of independence, reduced mobility, pain, and death. Consider these facts: *One in two women and one in five men will develop osteoporotic fractures. A woman's risk of developing a hip fracture is equal to the combined risk of developing breast, uterine, and ovarian cancer.*

While osteoporosis can be prevented and treated, there is, as yet, no cure. Prevention is the only way to avoid this disease and its debilitating consequences. Yet millions of Americans are not actively protecting themselves against osteoporosis. Over the past decade, we have slowly been uncovering important information about the causes of osteoporosis and ways to prevent it. One of the most significant findings is that osteoporosis is not an inevitable part of growing older. One of the great myths associated with this disease is that, as we age, we are all on our way to suffering hip fractures or becoming stooped over. This is a major misconception that causes individuals to overlook their risk and to avoid taking the necessary steps to prevent and treat osteoporosis.

7

Foreword

Osteoporosis develops silently over time. If I can convey just one thought to you, it is that it is never too late to prevent and/or treat osteoporosis. While it is true that we do not, as yet, have a cure for osteoporosis, there are steps you can take at every age to prevent and manage this disease. All along the way, from your teens through your twenties, to midlife and beyond, there are ways to promote your bone health and prevent osteoporosis.

The women's health movement has sent a powerful message to all of us about taking control of our health. We need to assess our risk for this disease and take personal action to prevent it or diminish its consequences. And we must step forward and demand that osteoporosis be advanced to a prominent place on the national health care agenda until a cure for the disease is found.

A recent report issued by the World Health Organization (WHO) states that the incidence of hip fractures, the most serious consequence of osteoporosis, is becoming a worldwide epidemic. WHO warns that if interventions are not implemented today, the disease will reach epidemic proportions early in the next century. Key steps to address this threat include an expanded federal research effort and a national education campaign to translate research findings into public health recommendations.

The National Osteoporosis Foundation is leading the way to support these significant research and education initiatives.

Foreword

Ruth S. Jacobowitz's timely and important new book, *150 Most-Asked Questions About Osteoporosis*, educates women on how to take control of their bone health and empowers them to seek the best possible health care in order to overcome this life-threatening and life-diminishing disease.

Sandra C. Raymond
Executive Director
National Osteoporosis Foundation

For Paul, then, now and always

Acknowledgments

This book is written for women—for all of us who are, I hope, not only going to live longer, but are going to live better. I believe we can, in fact, create our destiny when we learn the facts about diseases that can alter our life span. Osteoporosis, particularly postmenopausal osteoporosis, is one of those crippling diseases.

I am grateful to all the women, and men, who attend the seminars in which I participate and to all the health-care organizations that sponsor them. Their continuing commitment to and support of dispersing important information to consumers makes these kinds of vital programs possible. I am also indebted to the women and men who write to me and share their concerns and tell me their stories.

A special thank you to the physicians with whom I've shared the panels this past year: Mary K. Beard, Robert J. Bury, Charles H. Chesnut III, M. E. Ted Quigley, William D. Schlaff, and Sheldon A. Weinstein.

Acknowledgments

There are many other people who work hard for the success of these programs. I can't begin to name them all—I wish I could—but I thank them profusely.

I am also deeply appreciative of the assistance of Charles H. Chesnut III, M.D., professor of Medicine, Radiology, and director, Osteoporosis Research Center, University of Washington, and to Sandra C. Raymond, executive director of the National Osteoporosis Foundation, for reading the manuscript and for their important messages in this book.

To my editor, Toni Sciarra, at Hearst Books/William Morrow and Company—I can say sincerely, reflecting on the three projects we've done together—each book was improved by your creative input, your superb editorial skills, and your genuine friendship. A special thanks, too, to Tim Hazen at Hearst Books and to Laurie Gibson Lindberg, National Osteoporosis Foundation, who always gave their time and expertise to answering my questions.

My thanks to Marilyn Morgan, Iris Bailin, and Deanne Siegal, M.S., R.D. Your help was invaluable.

I think often of my mother, Claire Scherr, who has always considered exercise and healthful eating to be important. I thank my family, Harriet and Bud Lewis, Susan and Leonard Rosenberg, and Rifkie and Bill Jacobowitz, who over the years shared good-health stories with me—and snuck unhealthful snacks with me on occasion, too. I thank all my children and grandchildren: Jan Jacobowitz, Alvin and Jeffrey Asher Lodish; Jody, David, Claire Michelle, and Jake

Acknowledgments

Cremer Austin; and Julie, Lowell, and Michael Aaron Potiker, who never mind the time that the books and lectures take and who always express pride in what I am doing.

Yet, as always, it is to my husband, Paul, that I am most indebted for sharing with me a life so filled with love and companionship that I had the time and the mind to reach out to the larger world—and to try to help others.

Ruth S. Jacobowitz

Contents

Contents

Before You Begin This Book

Remember me? I'm the medical writer who fell headlong and unprepared into menopause and not only survived, but flourished. Then I began to tell and write about it. My book, *150 Most-Asked Questions About Menopause: What Women Really Want to Know*, was published in January 1993. Prior to that, I coauthored *Managing Your Menopause* with my physician, Wulf H. Utian, M.D., Ph.D., a world expert on menopause. Since its publication in 1990, I have been traveling around the country, lecturing on women's health issues. My goal was, and continues to be, to help inform and empower women so that they can handle menopause and other health issues smoothly and with a strong foundation of knowledge.

What happened when I, a medical journalist and former vice president of Mt. Sinai Medical Center in Cleveland, Ohio, unsuspectingly encountered menopause is what drives me to continue to write books and to lecture—an outgrowth of my need to try to ensure that what happened to me would not happen to any other woman—anywhere. I believe that we all need to educate ourselves, empower ourselves, and plan so that we can enjoy a first-rate second half of life.

I've had the opportunity to share my story with more than twenty thousand women in person and millions of others through the media. More important, I've listened to their stories and their questions and learned firsthand what women really want to know about menopause and other midlife issues.

This information, plus data from the first Gallup Poll ever undertaken to learn what women know (and feel they need to know) about menopause provided me with vital facts. I decided the best way to share it all with you was to give you a really useful, easy, perhaps even fun-to-read book that would deliver information in much the same way that it comes to me—through a large number of questions and answers salted with solid medical advice from experts, and peppered with amusing and insightful anecdotes collected on my travels. I studied the questions that women asked and reviewed more than ten thousand questionnaires that they had completed. Then I selected the one hundred and fifty most-asked questions about menopause.

Over the past year, I've visited Salt Lake City, San Diego, Minneapolis, Denver, Kansas City, Dallas, Pittsburgh, New York, Milwaukee, and other cities. I've been collecting more questions from the women at the programs, and this time their interests directed me toward focusing on answers to questions about osteoporosis. Osteoporosis is the most common and potentially the most debilitating bone disease in the world. It is characterized by the loss of bone mass, reducing the density and strength of bones, which leads to greatly increased risk of fractures. Osteoporosis literally means "porous bone."

Now that we women have the opportunity to live a full half of our adult life after menopause, many of us are asking more and more questions about osteoporosis and its power to disfigure, cripple, or kill us, and, more importantly, what can be done to prevent it. On the tour that I began in the fall of 1992, I found that women were much more interested in postmenopausal osteoporosis than they had been earlier, and that they asked many more questions about how to prevent, recognize, and treat it. Even as I write this book, I continue to lecture and listen to more women in more cities. And I continue to be struck by the ever-increasing numbers in which women come out to educate themselves on their own behalf and to eliminate medical myths for their own generations and for all time. I am also impressed by the number of men who are now in our audiences.

From these sources, I have selected the one hundred and fifty most-asked questions about osteoporosis for inclusion in this book. It is divided into sections such as: who is at risk;

how does menopause affect our bones; and what life-style changes can we make to protect ourselves and preserve our bone mass.

The programs from which these questions are drawn all follow a similar format. Guests are invited to the programs through the media or by flyers or invitations sent to them from the sponsoring medical organizations or institutions in their communities. The programs are held in the evening for the maximum convenience of the women who work and the ever-increasing number of men who accompany them.

In addition to the audience's most-asked questions about osteoporosis, this book shares the results of a 1991 National Family Opinion Survey of a thousand women ages forty to sixty, which tells us what still other women say they know or need to know about postmenopausal osteoporosis. Other surveys are included as well.

In *150 Most-Asked Questions About Osteoporosis: What Women Really Want To Know,* you'll learn about the kinds of bone-density testing available, what the tests reveal, which women are candidates for osteoporosis, and how women of all ages can "bone up" with the help of the right kinds of exercise, diet, calcium supplements, and hormone replacement therapy. We'll briefly review menopause, what it is, when it occurs, and how it can affect the health of our bones. I'll also present questions and answers about treatment for osteoporosis, tell you what women are saying and doing about osteoporosis, and include a risk-factor checklist to help you measure your risk and take action so that you can keep standing tall.

We're going to explore how women actually feel when they're told they've suffered bone loss and what they're doing about it. I'm also going to suggest new ways for packing calcium into your diet and describe the best bone-building exercises. So give up all of your formerly conceived notions about what midlife and beyond might look and feel like, and let's get ready to give ourselves a straight shot at the longest prime of life we can create!

It is important, however, not to see that lengthy prime of life as a way to chase after eternal youth. To every age there is a special quality that can be enhanced and enjoyed. I believe that the postmenopausal years can be the beginning of that extended prime of life. To quote a noted physiologist and teacher:

Boredom is our number one enemy; not the boredom of nothing to do, but the boredom of not doing anything that thrills and delights us.

> Estelle R. Ramey, M.D.
> Ph.D., professor emeritus,
> Georgetown University.

CHAPTER 1

What Is Osteoporosis?

I don't know who first called osteoporosis the "silent thief." I do think it is a perfect description of this disabling deficiency disease. I first heard of osteoporosis in the early 1980s, when I was still at Mt. Sinai. I clearly remember wondering whether this was a medical marketing invention. It seemed to appear on the medical writing scene so abruptly!

As consumers of health care, most of us became aware of osteoporosis only a dozen or so years ago. In fact, the National Osteoporosis Foundation (NOF), a nonprofit health organization dedicated to reducing the incidence of osteoporosis, was founded only recently, in 1986. NOF serves as the foremost resource for individuals and for health-care professionals who are seeking the most up-to-date, medically sound information about this disease. (Information about how to contact NOF can be found in Appendix D.)

The National Family Opinion Survey revealed that 95 percent of the women surveyed in 1991 had heard of osteoporosis, but knew little about it. Women closer to, at, or past, menopause showed a somewhat greater familiarity with the risk factors concerning osteoporosis. However, most of those surveyed did not know how many women over age forty-five get osteoporosis or that the condition can be a result of menopause.

The thousands of questionnaires I've been studying from the more recent consumer programs in which I participate indicate a growing awareness among women of the disabling effects of osteoporosis and, most recently, have begun to show a better understanding of risk factors and risk-factor intervention. Women are asking more questions about osteoporosis and bone-density tests and about nutrition, exercise, and calcium supplementation as they affect our bones. Women say they want more information about prevention and treatment.

In particular, women who have had a long family history of the disease are keenly aware that all the women in their families became "little women" as they aged. Losses in height of more than four inches were not uncommon. The "dowager's hump," that curvature of the upper back that medically is called dorsal kyphosis, was not uncommon in these families, either. At the programs, some of these women told me that before they learned that osteoporosis could be prevented, they thought that these changes in stature and in posture were just how their families aged. One woman from Kansas City said she simply thought that while in some families men and women lost some of their hair, people in her family lost some of their height.

Not so, although both changes can be the result of hereditary predisposition. However, the interesting positive fact about osteoporosis is that *this is one disease for which we can significantly alter our hereditary odds*. With osteoporosis, we can cut right across the matrix of our genetic programming, *if* we learn about and are willing to do something about it. It is never too soon to take an active role in protecting your bones.

A business acquaintance of mine who has become a fairly close telephone friend was fascinated when I told her that I was participating in programs about menopause and writing a book about osteoporosis. "Are you doing this for me?" she asked kiddingly. This friend—I'll call her Sydny—explained that her family history made her fear getting older. She told me of her aunt who at seventy continued to ice skate and who all her life had walked across the Brooklyn Bridge into Manhattan. Then one day, she tripped on a curb while crossing the street. She fell, her hip was fractured, and the X-ray revealed frail, porous bones that appeared to be disappearing. The hip never healed, and Sydny's aunt went to a nursing home. She died there, just one year after the accident, from pneumonia and infection—complications that frequently take the lives of elderly osteoporosis patients who are laid up with broken bones.

Syd also watched her mother gradually grow shorter; the

woman's upper vertebrae collapsed, until she seemed to have no neck. Her head jutted forward to compensate for the large "dowager's hump" on her upper back. Both Syd's mother and aunt had been rather short and sturdy women who were slightly overweight. Their stature, weight, and sturdy build did not protect them from the ravages of osteoporosis. Their risk factors included a family history of the disease, a lifelong deficiency in calcium intake, and an extended use of excessives doses of thyroid medication. (More about these risk factors and how they affect us will be covered in Chapter Three.)

Because of her family history, Syd knew early on that she had to protect her bones. She is on postmenopausal estrogen therapy, and she walks on her treadmill every morning for thirty minutes before she goes to work. She eats calcium-rich foods, which we'll discuss in Chapter Seven, and she takes calcium supplements. But she's still frightened. What happened recently to her tall, slim sister, Leslie, didn't help to allay her fears.

Syd's sister, Leslie, had been a fashion model in her younger years. All of her life, Leslie walked straight and tall, with that runway bounce and verve. She was still turning heads at the age of fifty-three—at least, she did until recently.

Just a few months ago, Leslie was baby-sitting for her grandson. When he toddled under a table, it began to tip as

28

if getting ready to fall upon him. Leslie jumped up, and she fell as she grabbed the baby out of harm's way. The baby was fine; Leslie's pain was excruciating. She had broken her breastbone. It was the X-rays, and the subsequent bone-density test, that alerted her doctors to the fact that she was in trouble—big trouble. Leslie had advanced osteoporosis.

In time, the breastbone fracture healed. Leslie took calcium supplements, ate properly, and exercised more than ever. Then one day as she sat at her desk, she swiveled around in her chair to reach her files. That simple, slow swivel fractured two ribs. Today Leslie is on calcitonin injection therapy (which is covered in Chapter Nine), and every morning she jumps to light rock music on her mini-trampoline. She told me that she is dedicated to doing whatever she can to halt the demineralization of her bones, and she is willing to try anything to rebuild bone, if that is possible. But she says wistfully, "How come no one knew how to help me avoid this when I was young?" You can be sure she is counseling her daughters and nieces now.

Syd and Leslie are women of the 1990s, women who know that they need to learn as much as they can if they want to beat the odds of a family history of a disease that no one talked much about until very recently. Today, much more is known about osteoporosis, and women tell me that they are ready to learn what osteoporosis is, what it does, and how they can work to improve their skeletal future.

1. WHAT IS OSTEOPOROSIS?

Osteoporosis is the most common and potentially the most debilitating bone disease known to man—and woman. Osteoporosis creates "porous bones." Sadly, more than twenty-five million Americans suffer from this disease; twenty million are women. The disease is marked by a loss of bone tissue, or bone mass, which also means a loss of bone strength. Statistics reveal that one-half of women over fifty will fracture a bone because of osteoporosis.

2. WHAT IS POSTMENOPAUSAL OSTEOPOROSIS?

The majority of women who get this disease have a form of it called postmenopausal osteoporosis: osteoporosis that shows up after their estrogen-production system has shut down. In fact, it is estimated that approximately one-third of all women over fifty will suffer a spinal, or vertebral, fracture in their later years.

3. WHAT CAUSES POSTMENOPAUSAL OSTEOPOROSIS?

Postmenopausal osteoporosis is caused by the rapid bone loss some women experience in the first seven to ten years after their last menstrual period. This is a disease with a progression that can be likened to the domino effect: Loss of bone mass leads to reduced bone strength, which leads to an increased risk of fractures.

4. HOW CAN OUR BONES BECOME POROUS?

Our bones are living tissue formed from a soft protein framework made up mostly of collagen. Healthy bones are constructed with an outer shell of dense bone, called *cortical bone*, that encases an internal structure of spongy-looking bone, called *trabecular bone*. The strength in our bones comes partly from calcium. In fact, approximately 99 percent of the calcium in our body can be found in our bones and in our teeth.

Now let's look at osteoporotic bone. In persons with osteoporosis, the cortical bone is no longer dense; it has become thin, like fine china. The internal trabecular bone looks like its spongy holes have been greatly enlarged. The bone holding this holey honeycomb structure together is thin and frail. These kinds of bones can fracture easily.

5. HOW MANY FRACTURES OCCUR EACH YEAR BECAUSE OF OSTEOPOROSIS?

Osteoporosis is responsible for more than 1.5 million fractures per year. Its economic impact exceeded ten billion dollars in the United States in 1990. The cost continues to escalate as our population ages. Yet, in the 1991 National Family Opinion Survey, less than 42 percent of the women surveyed believed that osteoporosis can be a result of menopause. This indicates that we women need to learn more about this disease.

6. WHY ARE SO MANY WOMEN AFFLICTED WITH OSTEOPOROSIS?

Almost all women build bone mass until the age of thirty to thirty-five. Then we usually begin to lose bone at about the rate of 1 percent per year. However, after menopause (without estrogen replacement therapy), for about seven to ten years, that rate accelerates to a loss of 3 percent or more of bone density per year. Just think of it: If we lose 3 percent of our bone per year for ten years, we have lost 30 percent of our bone mass. After these years of rapid bone loss, the loss levels off again to about the 1 percent per year that is typical of aging. However, by then we're already at a disadvantage vis-à-vis our bone mass.

7. DO MEN LOSE BONE AS THEY AGE, TOO?

Men lose bone as they age as well, but they lose it at approximately the same steady low rate of 1 percent per year, with no acceleration such as women experience. Men also have the additional protection of having heavier bone mass.

8. WHAT CAUSES THE DIFFERENCE IN BONE LOSS BETWEEN WOMEN AND MEN?

As women enter menopause, estrogen levels begin to drop, dwindle and, for most of us, disappear. Decreased estrogen levels in our bodies accelerate the bone loss that

has been part of our natural aging process and may lead us to develop osteoporosis. Estrogen plays a role in preserving a positive calcium balance in our bones by suppressing the rate of bone resorption (resorption is the process by which old bone is discarded). According to *Clinical Symposia* (Volume 39, 1987), a medical manuscript about osteoporosis by Frederick S. Kaplan, M.D., "The exac mechanism by which estrogen asserts its effect on bone unknown. No estrogen receptors have ever been found bone cells." Nonetheless, Dr. Kaplan writes, "It is cle however, that estrogen replacement therapy (ERT) is n effective in preventing Type I osteoporosis (postme pausal osteoporosis) in the *perimenopausal* period v rates of trabecular bone loss are the highest."

9. DON'T WE ALL LOSE AND GAIN BONE THROUGHOU LIVES?

Yes, bone is living and growing tissue. It is metabolically active. However, in our thirties, the process that we call *bone remodeling* can begin to unbalanced. Let's take a moment to review c natural bone-remodeling cycle. In *150 Most-A tions About Menopause*, I described the proces "There are voracious Pac-Man–like critters in called *osteoclasts*. They are programmed to 'go get rid of old bone in a process called resorptic

also worker-critters, called *osteoblasts*, whose job it is to busily build new bone tissue to replace the old." It is vital that the work of the builders stays ahead of the work of the gobblers, or soon we begin to lose bone tissue. Until we are in our thirties, that's no problem for most of us. The builders are ahead. Then, around the age of thirty-five, our balanced process changes and, if we do nothing to prevent it, the gobblers take the lead. (There are other circumstances in which we can lose bone even earlier, such as pregnancy or breast-feeding, if we do not accelerate our calcium intake. These are discussed in detail in Chapter Four.)

10. How do I know if I am at risk for osteoporosis?

The risk factors that may contribute to the development of osteoporosis are: a family history of the disease; an early menopause (usually thought to be before age forty-five); a small, thin stature; being Caucasian or Asian; having a sedentary life-style; having had a diet that was perpetually low in calcium; and taking medications that cause bone loss.

11. How much of my risk is hereditary?

Heredity is a major risk factor for osteoporosis. Interestingly, however, that's a risk factor that you can work toward modifying greatly if you begin early enough in your life to select a calcium-rich diet and to perform weight-

bearing exercises on a regular basis. Ideally, both these interventions would begin in your teen years and continue throughout your lifetime. But it's never too late to tamper with fate! I'll be discussing dietary calcium, calcium supplementation, and weight-bearing exercises in Chapters Six and Seven.

12. WHAT DOES POROUS, THINNING BONE LOOK LIKE?

On page 40, you can see a photograph of normal bone next to a photograph of thin, porous osteoporotic bone. Let's review the bone remodeling process: old bone is retired and new bone is added in a constant cycle. When more old bone is taken away than new bone is added, the bones begin to get larger holes in them, and our skeleton begins to look like a sponge that we might pick up in the ocean. Note in the osteoporotic bone photograph that in the "sea sponge" the holes are still connected by membrane, but the holes are larger and the connecting membrane is thinner, or finer. This is what we can envision when our doctors say that our bones are becoming more porous as we age.

13. WHAT CAN I DO NOW TO PREVENT OSTEOPOROSIS?

Good health and life-style habits that begin early in our lives can greatly minimize our risk for osteoporosis. Later in this book we're going to describe bone-building and bone-preserving, weight-bearing exercises, as well as plans for consuming an adequate amount of calcium-rich foods. But even before you get to those chapters, you can quit smoking (which speeds up menopause and, thus, the period of rapid bone loss) and you can start to limit your alcohol, which inhibits calcium absorption. Limiting caffeine and sodas is a healthy habit, too. (More about appropriate limits appears throughout the book.) Begin now and you'll be helping your bones and helping yourself.

14. I HAVE MANY OF THE RISK FACTORS FOR OSTEOPOROSIS. WHAT SHOULD I DO?

Discuss osteoporosis with your physician. The diagnosis of osteoporosis should be based on your doctor taking a complete medical history and giving you a thorough physical examination. Many physicians also believe that women should have a baseline bone-density test when they begin menopause, so that future changes can be compared to the past bone-density test. Many insurance companies do not cover this type of preventive medical testing, but I believe they should, and I think we should all work toward that outcome. Trying to repair or halt damage is much more expensive to the health-care delivery system than preserving healthy bone. In Chapter Four, I'll talk more about bone-density testing.

15. DOES ESTROGEN REPLACEMENT THERAPY (ERT) OR
    HORMONE REPLACEMENT THERAPY (HRT) HELP TO PRE-
    VENT POSTMENOPAUSAL OSTEOPOROSIS?

Premarin, the oldest and most widely prescribed
estrogen pill; Estrace and Ogen, other estrogen pills; and
Estraderm, the first and (as of this writing) the only
estrogen patch available in the United States, all have
been approved by the Food and Drug Administration
(FDA) for use in the prevention of postmenopausal
osteoporosis. This approval is particularly significant for
women who are at high risk for osteoporosis, based on the
risk factors described in the answer to Question 10.
Replacing the estrogen that we have lost with natural or
synthetic estrogen can slow the acceleration of bone loss
that begins at menopause. This is an issue you should
discuss with your physician. Together, based on your own
medical profile, you can determine if you are able to take
replacement estrogen. In the National Family Opinion
Survey, more than half of the women surveyed believed
that "taking estrogen was effective as a preventive for
osteoporosis." Actually, according to Charles H. Chesnut
III, M.D., director of the Osteoporosis Research Center at
the University of Washington Medical Center in Seattle,
"The *only* proven preventive for postmenopausal osteoporosis is estrogen replacement therapy" (emphasis
added). Should you wish to pursue nonhormonal therapy

for the prevention of osteoporosis, look at calcium, diet, and exercise in Chapters Six and Seven.

16. IF I WANT TO USE ESTROGEN REPLACEMENT THERAPY (ERT) OR HORMONE REPLACEMENT THERAPY (HRT) TO PREVENT OSTEOPOROSIS, HOW LONG WILL I HAVE TO CONTINUE TO TAKE THESE DRUGS?

Before we delve into the answer to this question, let's look briefly at the difference between ERT and HRT. ERT refers to the use of estrogen alone and is currently scientifically believed to be all that a woman whose uterus has been surgically removed needs to take if she and her doctor determine that she is a candidate for estrogen replacement therapy. HRT is the combination of estrogen and progestin that a woman with an intact uterus usually takes in order to prevent buildup of the lining of the uterus which can create a precancerous condition. It is the estrogen, however, that prevents osteoporosis. Your physician will undoubtedly evaluate your medical history, your risk factors, and your current medical status before prescribing either HRT or ERT for the prevention of osteoporosis. You and your physician should also discuss how long you should take HRT or ERT for that purpose.

17. I HAVE OSTEOPOROSIS AND AM ON ERT. HOW LONG WILL I NEED TO BE ON ESTROGEN?

What Is Osteoporosis?

Most scientific indications are that treatment would need to continue over several years, at least over the seven to ten years of accelerated bone loss that begins at menopause. Many studies suggest that ERT or HRT, once begun, should be a lifelong therapy.

For years, women have been left out of medical research, so there continues to be much that is unknown about the unique workings of our bodies. We complain about the lack of concrete answers to our medical questions—we have every right to complain! Yet osteoporosis is one disease that has been studied in which the risk factors are clear, prevention is possible if begun early enough, a diagnostic test is available, and some modalities of therapy are FDA-approved. This is one change in our bodies that we assuredly can work to counteract, in part or even in full. So let's take charge! We must manage our own preventive health care, because our health is too valuable a personal resource to abrogate its care to anyone other than ourselves.

The willingness to accept responsibility for one's own life is the source from which self-respect springs.

> Joan Didion
> Quoted in *The Last Word*, Carolyn Warner
> (Prentice Hall, 1992).

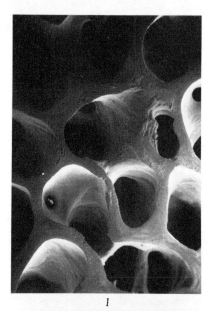

I

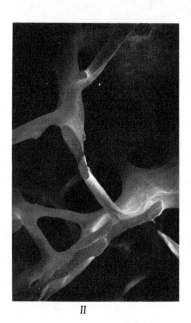

II

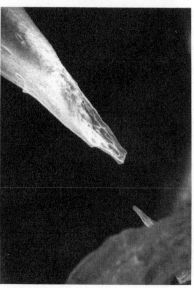

III

These are micrographs of biopsy specimens of normal and of osteoporotic bone. Photograph I shows normal bone from a seventy-five-year-old woman who does not have osteoporosis. Photograph II is from a forty-seven-year-old woman who has osteoporosis and has had multiple compression fractures. Photograph III shows a close-up of thin porous bone that has fractured.

From Dempster, D.W. et al., *Journal of Bone Mineral Research 1*, 15–21, 1986, with permission.

CHAPTER 2

How Do the Stages of Our
Lives Relate to Osteoporosis?

For those women and men who are thinking and reading about osteoporosis for the first time, a brief discussion of how our bones grow and remain strong through various ages and stages of our lives is important.

We are all born with a finite number of bones that make up our skeletons—206 bones, to be exact. Even though we add density to our bones, we grow no more new bones throughout our lifetimes, so we must take care of our bones to make sure they remain strong and can fulfill their vital functions.

Our bony skeleton permits us to be mobile, while supporting and protecting our total body. Throughout our lives, our calcium consumption and our weight-bearing exercise regimen permit our bones to remain strong. In the previous chapter, I described the necessary balance in our bone-remodeling process for bone maintenance. But let's go back now to our earliest years of childhood when our skeletons

41

grow because we add more bone tissue than we lose. That's how we grow!

When we become teenagers, our hormones play a role in this metamorphosis, and our bones are further strengthed by the production of our sex hormones. Androgen production in boys and estrogen production in girls brings about a surge in production of bone. Our bone growth is still ahead. Then we enter our twenties and thirties and, if our dietary and exercise habits promote good bones, our bone-remodeling process remains fairly balanced, although as early as in our twenties there can be some bone loss in the spine.

When we reach approximately age thirty-five, we have also reached our peak bone-mass development. That's the most bone mass we're ever going to have, and from then on, our job is to hang on to as much of our bone mass as we can. In subsequent chapters, this book is going to let you know how to do that and how to watch out for foods, medications, and life-style habits that can rob your bones of their strength.

Now we're moving along toward our forties and fifties, and assuming both women and men are engaging in life-styles that help to maintain as much bone as possible, we're all just losing bone at the rate of about 1 percent per year or less in the normal aging process. We're even, so far! Then along comes menopause, which speeds up bone loss significantly for women.

I think a brief discussion of menopause will be helpful so that we can understand its impact upon osteoporosis. First of all, menopause is neither a disease nor an illness. It is simply a transition: a bridge that women cross when we leave our reproductive selves behind and begin the nonreproductive half of our adult lives. It is a milestone like puberty, that transition that carried us from childhood into our reproductive teen years and the first half of our adult lives.

If you are wondering about the idea of two consecutive spans of adult life, let's look at those spans in mathematical terms. Women spend the first ten-to-thirteen-year span of their lives nonreproductively. Then from about age thirteen until approximately age fifty, which is about a thirty-seven-year span, most of us menstruate and can reproduce. We go through menopause at the average age of fifty-one years. (That simply means that we have gone twelve months without a menstrual period.) What happens next is an advantage of having lived in the twentieth century: If we are healthy at the age of menopause, according to medical statistics, we have a terrific chance of living to or beyond our mid-eighties. That's another thirty-seven years or so. That span is the second half of adult life that I've been talking about. It's the half with no more menstrual cramps and no more pregnancy worries. It's the half of adult life for some women in which they can really begin to do some of the things they always wanted to do but haven't had the time or financial ability to start. It's the time when they finally may have some time for themselves. For other women, who have chosen to defer childbearing until later in life, it offers the opportunity for the extra healthy years to raise younger families, provide for them, and see them grow. But this welcome opportunity for an increased life span presents us with a challenge—the challenge of taking care of ourselves and of protecting our own bodies. That's an appropriate, albeit weighty, responsibility.

Since we are planning to be responsible for making the most of those years, let's take a moment and review why menopause occurs and what it signals.

Remember that when we women are born, our ovaries contain all of the eggs that they will ever have: some half million. Once we pass through puberty and have our first period, we begin to lose eggs with each subsequent period. We never make any more eggs; we simply continue to use the abundant supply that is already in place within us.

Each month the pituitary gland, which is nestled in the base of the brain, sends out signals so that the female sex hormones, estrogen and progesterone, get ready to do their jobs, should a pregnancy occur. The estrogen makes the lining of the uterus lush, so it is ready to receive an egg that might be fertilized to create a life. If no fertilized egg materializes, along comes the progesterone that enables the uterus to shed that rich lining. And so the cycle continues, month after month.

When we have exhausted our lifetime supply of eggs, the estrogen and progesterone production slows down and finally, in most of us, shuts down altogether. That shutting-down process—with its various physical symptoms that affect many of us (such as those listed in the answer to question 25)—is known as menopause (although technically, menopause is defined only as our last menstrual period). Once we have gone a year without a period, we begin the postmenopausal period of our lives. Unless surgery intervenes, menopause is simply a natural transition that occurs around age fifty-one. Yet, some women may even stop ovulating every single month when they are still in their thirties. Menopause is as unique to each woman as her own experience of menstruation and pregnancy.

When she was in her late forties, my friend Trudy began to wonder if she was in menopause only after she realized that she hadn't had a period for a while and found herself thrusting first one arm and then a leg out from under the bed covers at night. When, in a sweaty flash, she threw off the covers altogether, she began to get suspicious. A check of the books in her library and a visit to her gynecologist confirmed her suspicion. Although she had chosen to ignore the first few missed periods, she learned from her reading and her subsequent doctor visit that her body was changing in many important ways. Many women tell me that they became aware of the beginning of menopause in much the same way.

When her revelation of menopause was confirmed, Trudy called me to say, "So, this is the beginning of menopause? I don't know if I'm going to like this. But, hormone replacement therapy—if I go on that, am I at risk for cancer? Maybe

I'll just live through this by sheer endurance. But what about the silent complication of menopause: osteoporosis and heart disease?"

Trudy's quandary echoes the confusion of most of us. How do we best prepare for the transition into that special second half of adult life? For many of us, our sexual fires are somewhat banked, although far from extinguished. Our tempers are tempered, reflecting our understanding of what is really important enough to us to make them flare! If we have mates, grown children, and grandchildren, they no longer take all our time and all our mind: We finally may have some delicious, guilt-free time for ourselves. We'll get into some of the issues for making that time prime time for all of us, including those women who still have children at home and still face school tuition and standing up at (and perhaps paying for) those children's weddings. But first let's define our terms: Let's make certain we understand menopause and the effect it can have on our skeletons and, thus, upon our lives.

18. WHAT IS MENOPAUSE?

As described above, menopause is simply the transition from our reproductive to our nonreproductive years. It may be caused at any age through having a hysterectomy with a bilateral oophorectomy (that means having the uterus and both ovaries removed). Whether natural or surgical, menopause signals the end of our reproductive lives. It indicates that our ovaries have slowed or stopped their production of estrogen.

19. WHY IS MENOPAUSE A MARKER FOR OSTEOPOROSIS?

The estrogen stoppage that occurs after menopause can accelerate our rate of bone loss from 1 percent per year to 3 percent or more per year in the first seven to ten years after menopause.

20. WHEN DOES MENOPAUSE OCCUR?

On average, women go through natural menopause at fifty-one years and four months of age. That hasn't changed much over the years. Women may go through natural menopause in their twenties or thirties, although that is thought to be rare. Or they may not go through menopause until their sixties. That is rare, as well.

21. I'M ONLY IN MY TWENTIES. WHY SHOULD I BE CONCERNED ABOUT MENOPAUSE AND ITS EFFECTS ON MY BONES? IT'S PROBABLY THIRTY YEARS AWAY.

I wish I'd had this book when I was in my twenties! But, alas, the scientific community didn't know then what it knows now. Now it is known that how we treat our bodies in our teens and twenties, in terms of calcium

47

consumption and exercise, can determine how straight and tall we live our lives and can directly affect our enjoyment of our golden years. This book is going to tell you how to achieve a sturdier skeleton no matter what your age, but its advice will be even more beneficial to you if you are still in your early-to-mid-thirties, since this is when most women usually achieve their *peak* bone mass.

22. WHAT IS SURGICAL MENOPAUSE?

Surgical menopause is the result of having a hysterectomy with a bilateral oophorectomy (the surgical removal of the uterus and both of the ovaries). This procedure ends our reproductive life in a much more incisive manner than the process of natural menopause, which occurs over a period of years. About 590,000 hysterectomies are performed in civilian hospitals in the United States each year. They are performed as a result of diagnoses of fibroids, endometriosis, uterine prolapse, pelvic inflammatory disease, and endometrial hyperplasia. Some critics of hysterectomy (which is the second-most-frequently performed surgical procedure on women, exceeded only by cesarean section) report that up to two-thirds of these procedures may be unnecessary. There are relatively few times when a hysterectomy is performed as emergency surgery. Inasmuch as time is in your favor, learn as much as you can about the procedure, try to save both your ovaries, if possible, and always seek a second opinion before you commit to surgery.

23. WHAT HAPPENS AFTER BOTH NATURAL AND SURGICAL MENOPAUSE THAT MAY BE HARMFUL TO MY BONES?

As we discussed earlier, when your ovaries run out of eggs (or are removed surgically), your body shuts down its estrogen and progesterone production system. Estrogen, one of the female sex hormones, helps to prevent osteoporosis by preserving the positive calcium balance in our bones, thereby slowing the rate of bone loss. How it actually does that is unknown. Experts still aren't sure how or if progesterone affects bone loss.

24. IF I HAVE NO MORE EGGS, WHY DO THE TWO FEMALE SEX HORMONES MATTER TO ME?

Therein lies the problem. Estrogen literally bathes and nourishes many organs and systems in our bodies. There are estrogen receptors (a place in a cell that can combine with and anchor estrogen to the cell) located throughout our bodies. Scientific research indicates that as many as three hundred different body processes can be affected by estrogen loss. Examples include loss of bladder control, short-term memory loss, and the thinning and drying of our tissues. So although estrogen may no longer be needed for its role in reproduction, for many of us its supporting roles, such as a maintainer of bone mass, begin to suffer.

25. WHAT ARE THE SYMPTOMS OF MENOPAUSE AND WHAT DO THESE CHANGES MEAN TO ME AND MY BONES?

The first signal of menopause is usually quirky changes in your menstrual periods. Your periods may get closer together, further apart, heavier, or lighter. This may go on for a long period of time. For some 75 percent of us, the hot flash is the first definite news we get about menopause. It and its twin, the night sweat, may be responsible for many of the other symptoms some of us may experience, such as palpitations, insomnia, disorientation, mood swings, anxiety, fatigue, and minor depression. Vaginal dryness and soreness make sex uncomfortable for some women after menopause. There is a long list of other changes that may occur as primary or secondary symptoms or as the outcome of our changing hormone levels at menopause. It is the silent and slow changes to the skeleton that are the subject of this book.

26. SO WHAT SHOULD I DO IF I THINK THAT I'M GOING THROUGH MENOPAUSE?

A visit to your physician with a list of your symptoms is a good way to find out if you are going through menopause. Once your doctor has taken a complete history and given you a physical examination, a simple blood test that reveals the serum estradiol (estrogen) concentration or the follicle-stimulating hormone (FSH) levels in your blood should provide the answer. Read all you can to learn more about menopause and osteoporosis and, with the help of your doctor, find out what these menopausal changes may mean to your bones. But don't despair; you can do something about preventing osteoporosis. In most cases, it's up to you!

27. I'VE HEARD A LOT ABOUT ESTROGEN AND PROGESTIN REPLACEMENT THERAPY. SHOULD I TAKE HORMONE REPLACEMENT THERAPY?

Figuring that out with the help of a doctor who really understands menopause and hormone replacement therapy (HRT) is very important to you at the time of natural or surgical menopause. Up to one-third of women may not need to take hormones for the early and uncomfortable symptoms—but, for those of us who do, hormone therapy can be very important. Estrogen may help us eliminate hot flashes, night sweats, and vaginal dryness, soreness, and irritation, as well as smooth out our mood swings, lessen our anxieties, stop our palpitations, enrich our sex lives, and enhance our sleep. However, for the long-term and potentially life-threatening diseases, such as osteoporosis and—if current studies under way are proven accurate—

heart disease, then perhaps we should all consider HRT or ERT, whichever is appropriate. There is more information about HRT and ERT in Chapter Eight.

I remember when I first knew something was changing in me. I was in my early forties when I had a hysterectomy, but my ovaries were intact, so I didn't get thrown into menopause. Without my uterus, however, I had no telltale seesawing of my menstrual periods to give me any clues as to why I was experiencing strange symptoms. I remember, too, that each time I mentioned what I thought were odd symptoms to my doctor, he said, "No, not menopause yet; you're just borderline." I was thrilled to be just borderline. Borderline what? Borderline young?

Later I realized that I was so caught up in being told, in effect, that I was still on the sunny side of menopause that I didn't bother to find out why I wasn't feeling up to par or why strange things were happening to me. Big mistake!

As I said earlier, I fell headlong into menopause and had the bad bumps to prove it. So I know all about denial. That's why I am so determined to make other women masters of their own health care. That's why I keep lecturing and writing and trying through education and information to empower other women to learn everything they can about this vital passage so they can make this trip to the second half of life with poise and equanimity.

I can't emphasize too strongly how important it is that you

learn all that you can about how our bodies age, that you not deny symptoms when they occur, that you adopt a life-style that promotes your good health, and that you find a physician who is interested in the ongoing care of women as we age and who is willing to be your partner in your quest to stay active and healthy.

The best-informed patient gets the best treatment.

> Isadore Rosenfeld, M.D.,
> cardiologist and author of
> *The Best Treatment*
> (Bantam, 1992), writing in
> *Vogue*, September 1992.

CHAPTER 3

Who Is at Risk for Osteoporosis? Am I a Candidate?

Sometimes I can't help seeing what appears to me to be the sign of osteoporosis. I can be going up the escalator in a shopping mall and see a woman just ahead of me with a slightly, or greatly, rounded back and I think—osteoporosis. Or, if I happen to glance over at the down escalator, which in some locations rides just next to the one going up, I notice a woman who is slightly or greatly stooped and whose chin seems to be too close to her chest, resting there almost without benefit of her neck, and I wonder if she has had her bone density tested for signs of osteoporosis. As more women live longer, I guess even more examples of osteoporosis will be easily sighted.

When I first began to speak at programs concerning menopause, there was little in the programs about osteoporosis other than the fact that it was a disease that we women could prevent or at least halt through life-style changes and, perhaps, by taking estrogen or combined hormone therapy.

Who Is at Risk for Osteoporosis? Am I a Candidate?

Today, however, a full third of most of the programs in which I am engaged are devoted to a discussion of osteoporosis and its detection and prevention. Today, we know that almost as many women die each year from osteoporosis-related illnesses as die from breast cancer. So in just one decade, public health officials and the National Osteoporosis Foundation have pinpointed osteoporosis as a major health problem.

And a major health problem it is! Just think of this: If a woman is healthy in her fifties, she will probably live well into her eighties, yet one woman in two will experience a fracture caused by some degree of osteoporosis by the time she is sixty-five! So why did such an insidious disease that is so common in middle and old age take until so late in the twentieth century to attract medical, media, and public attention?

First of all, osteoporosis is a complicated disease and little research was done earlier. Second, its cause is not completely understood, and its treatment is neither fully agreed upon nor assured, even now. Today, it stands fourth on the list of the National Institutes of Health as a leading cause of death of women—following heart disease, cancer, and stroke. Death from osteoporosis is usually as a result of complications that may follow bone fractures. Can you even begin to imagine the 1.5 million bone fractures a year that cause discomfort, disability, and even death? Think of the more than quarter-million hip fractures a year from which half of the women will never be able to walk independently again, of the 30 percent of these who will become totally dependent, and of the 15 to 20 percent who will spend the rest of their lives in nursing homes. Consider the 12 to 20 percent of women who die from pneumonia and blood clots, the complications that can follow within six months after the fracture.

So the question to be answered remains: Are you at risk?

28. HOW DO I FIND OUT IF I AM AT RISK FOR OSTEOPOROSIS?

In order to learn your risk for osteoporosis, consider your answers to the following questions and be assured that an explanation of the questions and answers follows later in this chapter:

Are you a thin, small-boned female?
Are you age forty-five or older?
Are you Caucasian or Asian?
Do you have a family history of osteoporosis?
Do you smoke?
Do you exercise?
Do you drink more than two ounces of alcohol a day?
Does your diet contain fewer than one thousand milligrams of calcium per day?
Have you gone through menopause?

Do you regularly take medications that may leach calcium from your bones, such as corticosteroids, excessive amounts of thyroid supplements, or antacids that contain aluminum? (More about this in the answer to Question 49, later in this chapter.)

Do you imbibe an excessive amount of caffeine?

Do you drink more than one or two sodas each day?

The above are all risk factors for osteoporosis. I'll explain how they can affect your risk in the answers to the questions in this chapter. There are no right or wrong answers to these questions, just *your* answers, which you should share with your physician so that you can begin to understand whether or not you are a candidate for this disease.

29. IF, ACCORDING TO THE QUIZ, I AM AT RISK, WHAT CAN I DO NOW?

Perhaps now is the time for you to have your bone mass measured and to begin a lifelong set of life-style changes in order to eliminate, or at least limit, your risk. Even if you have a genetic basis for being at risk, you can work to offset your genetic programming by consuming a calcium-rich diet, doing weight-bearing exercise, and eliminating substances that are harmful to you.

Even if you already show signs of osteoporosis, you can

usually work successfully toward stopping it in its tracks. In fact, the most compelling questions at our programs concern halting the progress of this disease. Yet 85 percent of the women who filled out our questionnaires at the conclusion of the program indicated that they had never had a bone mass measurement test for osteoporosis. This statistic is representative of most cities from which I have studied questionnaire results.

Information on what kinds of bone-density tests are available can be found in Chapter Four. Later chapters explore the pros and cons of drugs for the prevention and treatment of osteoporosis.

30. WHY IS THE BONE RESORPTION PROCESS DIFFERENT IN WOMEN THAN IN MEN?

It isn't. It works much the same way. Women's greater risk of getting osteoporosis has to do with two factors. First of all, women often have less bone mass to begin with than men, so that even though both lose bone at the same general rate, men start out with heavier bones. Second, there is nothing in the male physiology to compare with menopause and the (usually) complete loss of a hormone. When women lose estrogen, their rate of bone loss increases from 1 percent per year to about 3 percent per year or more in the seven to ten years immediately following menopause. Men continue along at the same 1 percent per year of loss. Women rejoin that rate after their years of rapid bone loss, but it's a smaller skeleton combined with heavy postmenopausal bone loss that puts women at greater risk of osteoporosis than men.

31. I DRINK ABOUT A DOZEN DIET SOFT DRINKS EACH DAY. HOW DOES THIS AFFECT THE MINERALS IN MY BONES?

Like balancing bone loss against bone replacement, the answer to this question has to do with another body-system balancing act—that of balancing calcium and phosphorus. An optimum equilibrium point would be having two-and-one-half times as much calcium in your body as phosphorus. Well, soft drinks, all kinds of soft drinks—those with and without sugar or caffeine—are high in phosphorous, which can unbalance our systems and cause a calcium deficiency, which is a risk factor for osteoporosis.

If you consume too much phosphorus (as in soft drinks), the excess spills into your bloodstream. There, chemical signals get crossed as the phosphorous binds with calcium and makes it unavailable for your body's needs. Your body, sensing that the calcium is not available, sends for more and through a complex signal from the parathyroid gland to its hormone, takes the calcium that your body needs—from your bones!

59

32. RATHER THAN GIVING UP SODA, CAN'T I JUST TAKE ADDITIONAL CALCIUM?

The answer to this frequently asked question is *no*. Taking more calcium to offset the effect of too many soft drinks just won't work, because too much calcium can become toxic. Too much phosphorus can unbalance other minerals that you need in your body, such as copper, zinc, magnesium, and manganese. Don't start a battle of elements in your body, or your bones will be the losers.

33. HOW MUCH IS TOO MUCH CALCIUM?

Some experts say that you can exceed the Recommended Daily Allowance (RDA) of 1,000 milligrams of calcium for premenopausal women and women on ERT or HRT by 200 milligrams. Postmenopausal women not on ERT or HRT should stay at 2,000 milligrams. Excess calcium in our blood can lead to excess calcium in our urine, which may cause kidney stones. This can be painful and may damage our kidneys.

34. I AM USED TO DRINKING ABOUT SIX OR SEVEN DIET SODAS EACH DAY. WHAT DO I DO NOW?

It would be best if you severely limited your intake of sodas and colas (to one or two per day). Learn to drink water. It's so good for you. A daily intake of eight 8-ounce glasses of plain water can do wonders. It flushes toxins out of our systems, helping us to maintain our good complexions; it is a great dietary aid encouraging us to eat less and helping us to digest our foods better; it aids our elimination process and helps other bodily functions and systems to work better.

35. MY DENTIST REPORTS A SHIFTING IN MY TEETH AND HAS SUGGESTED A BONE-DENSITY TEST. CAN YOU EXPLAIN THE RELATIONSHIP BETWEEN TEETH AND BONES?

One of the first places that osteoporosis may show up is in the mouth. It is not uncommon for your dentist to be the first person who spots a change in bone health—sighting it in the density and strength of the jaw bone, which should hold your teeth firmly in place. Usually labeled "periodontal disease," which can include everything that happens in the mouth, osteoporosis may first be sighted as pyorrhea, gum disorders, or, as it actually is called, osteoporosis of the mouth.

If the bone in your jaw has become porous, as it would be in osteoporosis, it has also become less able to hold your teeth firmly in place. If your teeth begin to shift, your gums may become inflamed and may recede, opening the path for bacteria and infection.

No, don't panic. Tooth or gum problems aren't sure signs of osteoporosis, but they do bear checking into. Periodontal disease is the major cause of tooth loss as we age, and it is more common in women than in men. If you have some form of it, check it out. Find out whether you're dealing with a dental hygiene problem or an early signal of bone loss.

36. I AM A RECENTLY DIAGNOSED DIABETIC. DOES DIABETES CAUSE BONE LOSS?

Diabetes is a hormone-deficiency disease in which the hormone insulin is not secreted at normal levels in the body, and sugar is not metabolized as it should be. There does appear to be a correlation between the high sugar level in the blood of diabetics and osteoporosis. Long-term uncontrolled diabetes may lead to a significantly higher rate of osteoporosis in both female and male diabetics. This relationship has been known since 1948, but its scientific basis is not clearly understood. It appears that calcium absorption is depressed by the high sugar level. This could also result from the fact that both medical problems may be hereditary and, thus, a genetic link could exist. Or osteoporosis could be a result of the effect of insulin injections on bone resorption. In any event, it appears that diabetic women and men may have as much as 10 percent less bone mass than nondiabetics. This, coupled with the loss of the hormone estrogen, which is known to help prevent osteoporosis, may put postmenopausal women with diabetes at greater risk for osteoporosis. This is a subject that you should discuss in detail with your physician.

37. MY MOTHER HAS OSTEOPOROSIS THAT WAS DIAGNOSED LATE IN HER SEVENTIES. SHE IS A PETITE WOMAN, A NATURAL REDHEAD. I AM TALL AND RATHER BIG-BONED, LIKE MY FATHER. WILL I NECESSARILY INHERIT HER PREDISPOSITION TO OSTEOPOROSIS?

As we have described, heredity is one of the risk factors for osteoporosis. Each of us inherits a genetic tendency that will determine to a certain extent the size and strength of our bones. And science tells us that if our mothers had osteoporosis, our chances of getting it are greater. Yet osteoporosis is one of the diseases for which, with excellent early intervention, you can alter the hereditary factor. First of all, your body frame seems to be quite different from your mother's. Is your life-style different as well? For example, did your mother eat calcium-rich foods, perform weight-bearing exercises, abstain from smoking, and limit alcohol? Do you? Did she (or do you) take medications, like cortisone, that can retard calcium absorption? These and other questions should be raised by your physician, whom you should contact for a checkup. Your doctor may suggest a bone-density test, the findings of which may help to put your mind at ease. Your doctor also may prescribe the life-style changes that can begin to limit your risk.

38. DOES THE EARLY START OF MENSTRUATION CONTRIBUTE TO BONE LOSS?

The long bones in our body begin to fuse at the time of our first menstrual period. That is because the skeletal and reproductive systems work in harmony to guide our physical and sexual characteristics. So with early menstruation (or menarche, as it is medically named), our bones are set in terms of their length. Then an ongoing harmonious relationship between our pituitary gland and our ovaries exists, enabling us to produce the female sex hormones that help to keep our bones strong. So, yes, early menstruation sets your long bones, but it does not determine your bone strength or your risk of osteoporosis.

39. HOW DOES A LOSS OF OUR MENSES WEAKEN OUR BONES?

In several important studies conducted by Barbara Drinkwater, Ph.D., Department of Medicine, Pacific Medical Center in Seattle, it was demonstrated that women marathon runners who work out intensely enough to stop their menstrual periods (a condition called amenorrhea) are at risk for osteoporosis because of estrogen loss.

40. IS THE RISK OF OSTEOPOROSIS GREATER IN WOMEN WHO HAVE NOT HAD CHILDREN?

Some statistics do show that women who have given birth are less likely to show signs of osteoporosis than women who have never had children. It appears that the increased estrogen levels during pregnancy make women who have had a number of pregnancies less vulnerable to osteoporosis. These statistics, however, may be skewed by other factors such as individual hormonal functions, heredity, and even some social or environmental factors.

Women give up calcium to their children's bones during pregnancy and for as long as they nurse their infants. Whether they build or lose bone as a result depends upon their nutrition during and immediately after the pregnancy. Historically, symptoms of osteoporosis seldom surfaced during pregnancy, because women who were young enough to be pregnant usually were not old enough to experience osteoporosis. That is changing somewhat in the last decade or so with the increasing incidence of late pregnancies. It is important that you know that the Recommended Daily Allowance (RDA) for calcium increases during pregnancy and breast-feeding. Since most of us probably were not meeting our need for calcium prior to pregnancy, we may even need to *triple* our former calcium intake for maximum benefit during this time. For most women who don't take in enough extra calcium to meet the demands of pregnancy and nursing, our bodies respond by giving up the calcium from our own bones to meet those demands. Then our hormones rush out to help meet these needs by encouraging our systems to replace lost calcium more quickly.

41. I AM GOING THROUGH MENOPAUSE AT AGE THIRTY-FOUR. AM I AT A GREATER RISK FOR OSTEOPOROSIS THAN I WOULD BE IF MY BODY HAD WAITED UNTIL I WAS FIFTY?

Yes, you are, because you have stopped producing estrogen many years earlier than the average age range. Therefore, many of your body's systems, including your bones, will be deprived of the beneficial effects of estrogen for a longer period of time. Menopause is a good time to get back into the health-care delivery system, if you have not already done so, and to talk to your physician about calcium supplementation, hormone replacement therapy, and other life-style changes that can protect your bones.

42. I'M A MARATHON RUNNER, AGE TWENTY-SEVEN. I WAS DELIGHTED, AT FIRST, WHEN MY MENSTRUAL PERIODS DISAPPEARED ALONG WITH MOST OF MY BODY FAT WHILE I WAS IN TRAINING. NOW, MY DOCTOR TELLS ME THAT I AM EXPERIENCING AMENORRHEA (THE LOSS OF PERIODS). SHE SAYS I AM IN DANGER BECAUSE THE SLOWING DOWN OF ESTROGEN PRODUCTION IN WHAT

Who Is at Risk for Osteoporosis? Am I a Candidate?

SHE CALLS MY "EXCESSIVELY LEAN BODY" IS STARVING MY BONES. IS THAT TRUE?

Your doctor is right! When you exercise enough to stop your periods, you have changed the balance of your hormones. Women at greatest risk for osteoporosis are those who have experienced prolonged periods of diminished estrogen. Remember, estrogen directly affects as many as three hundred different body processes. Among other things, it encourages our bones to maintain their equilibrium in the bone-remodeling process—putting bone back in the same proportion that is destroyed. Without estrogen, bone is being lost and is not being replaced. This imbalance causes a negative balance in your bone bank. It is important that you work with your doctor to reverse this situation, bring back your periods, and encourage normal bone remodeling. A bone-density test might also be a good idea, so that you can see exactly what your bone density is in relation to where it ought to be. If you caught this situation early, I hope you will be able to reverse it in short order. Perhaps a change in your diet, with the addition of calcium-rich foods, additional calcium, or hormone supplementation may help as well. Obviously, as a marathon runner, you're not short on weight-bearing exercise, and I hope you don't smoke, or use alcohol excessively. It's time to get busy to work toward stimulating your estrogen

67

production, bringing back your periods, and protecting your bones.

43. ARE CREAKING, AND SOMETIMES PAINFUL, JOINTS A SYMPTOM OF BONE LOSS? WHAT CAN I DO TO STOP THE SYMPHONY OF MY JOINTS?

No, creaking joints are not a symptom of bone loss and osteoporosis is not a joint disease. But I am beginning to believe that creaking bones and other forms of joint pain are among the least-researched complaints of women at midlife. Studies show that between one-third and one-half of the women surveyed complained of either creaking or painful joints. This common problem frequently presents itself with, or even before, the first hot flash. Troubling joints seem to be related to a reduction of cortisone, a substance naturally secreted by our adrenal glands to keep our joints moving freely. It seems odd, but our exercise activity levels do not seem to influence whether or not we will experience joint discomfort. Check out painful or creaking joints with your physician to assure yourself that you do not have an underlying chronic medical problem, such as fibromyalgia (an arthritis-related, painful condition), arthritis, or osteoarthritis. Once your physician has ruled out these problems, you might want to consider extra vitamin B_6 (approximately 50 milligrams daily), vitamin E (400 International Units daily), or vitamin C and cod-liver oil (vitamin D), which, while not scientifically proven, many women do tell me works to alleviate painful and creaking joints. Other women report that they have just waited out the problem, and, for some, it simply disappeared. While waiting, you might want to begin a program of gentle stretching of the muscles around the joints to reduce the stress or tension on them.

44. WHEN I'M INJURED, I GET LIGAMENT AND TENDON STRAINS, RATHER THAN FRACTURES. DOES THAT MEAN THAT MY BONES ARE STRONG?

No. Perhaps you are just lucky that you have not fractured a bone when injured. If you are seeking reassurance that your bones are strong, I would suggest that you consider having a baseline bone-density test. More information about the types of bone-density testing can be found in Chapter Four.

45. I HAVE CRACKED SEVERAL RIBS IN THE LAST COUPLE OF YEARS. IS THIS A WARNING OF BONE-DENSITY LOSS?

It could be. If I were you, I would find out by having my bone density tested and discussing the cracking-ribs problem in detail with my physician. If you are lucky enough to get a warning of an impending or existing problem, heed that warning.

46. IS THERE A RELATIONSHIP BETWEEN ARTHRITIS AND OSTEOPOROSIS?

No, because arthritis is a joint disease and osteoporosis is a bone disease. Arthritis is an aggregate term, representing many kinds of conditions and diseases. In its more appropriate and narrow usage, it refers to abnormalities in the joints of our body, yet it also reflects a number of other conditions, *but it does not relate to osteoporosis*. The most common form is called osteoarthritis, a condition that usually worsens slowly with age and can start out so mild that its effects are undetectable for many years. Osteoarthritis most often is seen as an enlargement, or thickening, of the bone of the joint. We can see it most easily in the enlargement of the joints of the fingers, yet the most serious form of osteoarthritis is usually in the knee and hip joints.

Although osteoarthritis may be disabling, it is not related to osteoporosis. Interestingly, people with this form of arthritis often have very different body types from people with osteoporosis. People with severe osteoarthritis tend to be larger, both in muscle build and in the amount of weight they carry. People with osteoarthritic hips rarely break their hips. Osteoarthritic growth is usually hard and thick. People with osteoporosis, in contrast, are frequently smaller in build, stooped, and their bones, upon observation, are porous and frail.

People who have osteoarthritis must still be concerned about calcium consumption and exercise, and often joint-replacement surgery is performed to keep them active.

Rheumatoid arthritis is a different story. This is a crippling joint disease that is diagnosed by a blood test. People with rheumatoid arthritis tend to have more serious problems with osteoporosis than people in the general population. They often have less calcium circulating in their bloodstreams; they frequently are more sedentary because of their painful joints (thereby not building bone mass); they often take pain medications, such as cortisone-like drugs, which block calcium absorption, and thus, they break their hips and other bones more often.

There are also other less common types of arthritis. Like rheumatoid arthritis, these are often found in people with osteoporosis. The immobility and the medications used to treat arthritis can contribute to the development or progression of osteoporosis. The only form of arthritis that does not usually have a negative impact upon osteoporosis is osteoarthritis.

47. DOES LIVING WITH A HEAVY SMOKER INCREASE MY CHANCES OF OSTEOPOROSIS?

I can find no studies showing the effect of passive smoke on the bone-mineral content of the nonsmoker's body. There are many studies that indicate smoking brings on an earlier menopause, that menopause usually ends estrogen production, which has a negative effect on the maintenance of bone mass. Perhaps after more studies are done on the deleterious effect of passive smoke (a fairly new avenue of research), you'll be able to persuade that heavy smoker with whom you live to kick the habit. Until then, I wish that person would quit for his or her own good health!

48. I HAVE AN UNDERACTIVE THYROID GLAND AND FOR MANY YEARS HAVE TAKEN A DRUG CALLED SYNTHROID TO REPLACE MY DEFICIENCY OF THYROID HORMONE. DOES THIS PUT ME AT RISK FOR OSTEOPOROSIS?

There is little disagreement that thyroid hormone production can affect bone metabolism. An underactive thyroid gland, a condition called hypothyroidism, is usually treated with a drug such as Synthroid, which can literally "knock out" your own thyroid gland's production system, by replacing it. In doing so, if the levels are not right it can have the same effect on your system as if you were hyperthyroid, that is, secreting too much thyroid hormone, which is scientifically known to put you at a higher risk for osteoporosis. A simple, fairly new blood test, the Ultra Sensitive TSH (Thyroid Stimulating Hormone), can let your physician know whether the dose you're taking is right for you. If you are taking the correct amount of thyroid hormone replacement, bone loss shouldn't be a problem.

49. WHAT OTHER MEDICATIONS CAN CAUSE BONE LOSS?

Certain other categories of helpful drugs can, as a side effect, cause us to lose bone increasing our risk of developing osteoporosis by interfering with the balance in our bone-remodeling system. Corticosteroids are culprits. Used to reduce inflammation and as immunosuppressive agents, they are widely used to treat asthma, arthritis, lupus erythematosus, osteoarthritis, and other conditions. Aluminum-containing antacids may be harmful to your bones. When aluminum is present, extra calcium is excreted from your body because the aluminum combines with the body's phosphorus and the calcium, drawing them into your urine. This loss of calcium can weaken your bones. Aluminum also deposits in bones, causing osteomalacia (a softening of bones). Other drugs that can interfere with the health and strength of our bones include those that treat certain cardiac irregularities or prevent seizures, such as phenytoin and barbiturate anticonvulsants; methotrexate, a drug used in cancer and immune disorders; cyclosporine A, a drug used following organ transplantation; and gonadotropin-releasing hormones, often used to treat endometriosis. There are other prescribed medications and over-the-counter preparations that can harm your bones as well. Discuss your risk of osteoporosis with your doctor. Perhaps a bone-density test should be done for you. If you are at risk for losing bone and you are postmenopausal, maybe estrogen replacement therapy plus extra calcium and exercise should be considered.

This chapter began by asking, "Who is at risk for osteoporosis?" and "Am I a candidate?" How about taking the National Osteoporosis Foundation quiz on the next page to see where you stand? Just answer the following questions:

ARE YOU AT RISK FOR OSTEOPOROSIS?

QUESTION	YES	NO
1. Do you have a small, thin frame, or are you Caucasian or Asian?	☐	☐
2. Do you have a family history of osteoporosis?	☐	☐
3. Are you a postmenopausal woman?	☐	☐
4. Have you had an early or surgically induced menopause?	☐	☐
5. Have you been taking excessive thyroid medication or high doses of cortisonelike drugs for asthma, arthritis, or cancer?	☐	☐
6. Is your diet low in dairy products and other sources of calcium?	☐	☐
7. Are you physically inactive?	☐	☐
8. Do you smoke cigarettes or drink alcohol in excess?	☐	☐

The more times you answer "yes," the greater your risk for developing osteoporosis. See your physician, and contact the National Osteoporosis Foundation for more information (see Appendix D). Used with permission of the National Osteoporosis Foundation.

CHAPTER 4

~

What Kinds of Tests Can Tell Me If I'm Suffering Bone Loss?

Remember how we were always "boning up" on something for school, for work, or just studying something that interested us? For example, very recently I had to "bone up" on sports, since my grandson Jeffrey turned eight and into a sports enthusiast. How else could I communicate with him?

"Boning up" in terms of skeletal health ideally should begin when we are small children. Mary K. Beard, M.D., coauthor of *Menopause and the Years Ahead* (with Lindsay Curtis, M.D.), is a noted Salt Lake City obstetrician and gynecologist with whom I've shared the podium at programs in Minneapolis, Denver, and Salt Lake City. She often refers to osteoporosis as "a childhood disease," explaining that it is in childhood that the seeds for the disease may be sown. She usually shows a slide of two beautiful young girls, about age six or seven, at play. Dr. Beard explains: "Children are bone-builders, and they build bone, not only through childhood, but into their teenage years and up to about their

76

mid-thirties—so we know how important milk and calcium intake are." But what of the children who do not like milk and milk products, or who have allergies to them? They need to be given regular amounts of calcium-rich foods and, sometimes, various forms of calcium supplementation.

Providing enough calcium to young children is the concern of physicians and, of course, parents. That concern grows deeper as many young girls grow into teenagers who are worried about staying ultra-thin. Then the problem of getting enough calcium worsens. Many teenage girls and young female adults give up dairy products to "save calories," when they can simply switch to nonfat milk and nonfat yogurt. What a shame! They miss the opportunity during these valuable years to build peak bone mass.

Some women in their reproductive years are not aware that pregnancy can exact a toll on their bones. Women need to know that they may build, maintain, or lose bone as they share their own calcium with their babies throughout pregnancy and breast-feeding. During those times, women should be consuming extra calcium, because the sharing of calcium with their unborn child, and, then with their infant, raises their needs to 1,200 milligrams of calcium per day. Nutritionally, here again, it's up to women to choose whether they'll build or lose their bone mass!

Each of us has our peak bone-mass level predetermined genetically. Yet if we interfere with reaching that peak when we are young, as may happen through excessive dieting or through depletion during pregnancy and breast-feeding, we will not enter our postmenopausal years with our maximal bone mass. Numerous definitive medical studies have shown that the most rapid decline in bone mass occurs within the first ten years after menopause. Remember, both men and women lose bone mass as they age about 1 percent per year, but this number increases to 3 *percent per year* or more for women in the early postmenopausal years. If a woman loses 30 percent of her bone density during the first ten years after menopause, she will be at risk for developing fractures. By age eighty-five, a woman may have lost even more than the 30 percent of the bone mass she had at menopause. Some women may have even greater bone loss than that.

What that means to each of us is that one out of two women will sustain fractures after the age of fifty. If a woman is in her sixties, those fractures are likely to be of the wrist, ankle, or vertebra. In her eighties, they may be of her hip. One-half of the women who suffer hip fractures may never fully recover or walk independently again, and one-third may become totally dependent. Between 15 and 20 percent of them will die in the first six months from complications such as infection or pneumonia.

In Chapter One you learned that being Caucasian or Asian is a risk factor for osteoporosis. That risk stacks up as follows: African-American women have one half the risk and Hispanic women about one-third the risk of white and Asian women.

What Kinds of Tests Can Tell Me If I'm Suffering Bone Loss?

So, how do you learn where you are in terms of bone mass? How do you find out if you are one of the women who is entering menopause—and the years of rapid bone loss which are just beyond—with low bone mass? Did you take the National Osteoporosis Foundation's risk-factor test on page 75? How did you rate? In addition to those factors, physicians also believe that people who drink excessive amounts of alcohol, coffee, or soda will lose calcium throughout the day through their kidneys. They suggest keeping those "calcium depleters" to one or a maximum of two a day.

On the thousands of questionnaires that women completed at the programs, when asked if they had ever had a bone-screening test for osteoporosis, fewer than 15 percent so indicated. However, when asked if they were considering asking their physicians about the appropriateness of a bone-density test for them, more than 25 percent said "yes." Now, with that information at hand, perhaps you should ask your physician if he or she recommends a bone-density test for you.

50. WHAT IS A BONE-DENSITY TEST?

It is a test that will determine the bone-mineral density in a site in your skeleton and determine your risk of osteoporosis and fracture. According to Myron Winick, M.D., emeritus professor of nutrition, Columbia University

College of Physicians and Surgeons, writing in *Menopause Management* (November/December 1992), "A postmenopausal patient's risk for osteoporosis should be assessed not only by family history and other history-related indicators, but also by two bone-density measurements at six-month intervals. If bone loss is demonstrated in the tests, then estrogen replacement therapy (ERT) should be considered."

Since excessive loss of bone mass is the chief characteristic of osteoporosis, bone-density tests measure bone mass to ascertain how much bone loss has occurred. There are a number of different tests that measure different sites in the body, such as the spine, hip, or wrist. Your physician will undoubtedly determine which test is appropriate for you. These are not the traditional X-rays with which we are familiar, but rather tests that specifically measure bone mass using a photon or X-ray energy source to provide information.

Called bone densitometry, these tests are available in many health-care institutions and in some physician's offices. They assess changes in the bone for diagnostic purposes or to monitor the course of therapy for women who have already been diagnosed as having suffered bone loss. Many physicians consider bone densitometry an important test in determining whether a woman needs to take estrogen to preserve her bone mass. At this time, however, physicians do not consider densitometry mandatory for all women.

51. ARE THERE ANY OTHER KINDS OF TESTS TO DETERMINE BONE LOSS?

No. There are some blood and urine tests that can identify changes in blood or urine calcium content, which can show the rate of bone turnover to identify or rule out other diseases. The blood tests are more likely to be used to determine whether changes in bone are caused by some other disease, such as certain kinds of arthritis or bone marrow disease. Urine tests are not usually used to identify osteoporosis, but they may be used to study the efficacy of the treatment for osteoporosis.

52. ARE BONE-DENSITY TESTS PAINFUL? HOW LONG DO THEY TAKE?

There are a number of testing procedures, all of which are painless and noninvasive. Although different types of densitometry measure different places in the body, they are fundamentally the same in terms of how they work: An energy source derived from a photon (a particle of electromagnetic radiation) is passed over the wrist, hip, spine, or any other part of the skeleton in which the bone mass is being measured. The types of equipment used for the tests differ, and most take under fifteen minutes.

53. WHAT IS THE DEXA TEST?

DEXA refers to the newest, fastest, most precise, and most widely used technique for measuring bone. DEXA (Dual-Energy X-ray Absorptiometry) uses two beams of X-ray to measure structure deep within soft tissue, such as the hip and the spine or even the total body. The entire procedure takes about five minutes. DEXA exposes the patient to one-sixth the radiation of a routine chest X-ray, and far less than full dental X-rays. Moreover, it exposes the patient to a slightly lower radiation level than that of similar bone-density testing techniques, which are discussed in answers to the next few questions.

Let me describe how my DEXA test was performed. I was asked to lie on the procedure table on my back. A large square bolster was placed under my legs, just below my buttocks, so that my legs curved over the bolster. I was offered a pillow for my head. The radiologic technician who did my test asked me a number of questions concerning my risk factors and my life-style. Then, she asked me to refrain from moving the lower half of my body, and began the actual test. As the arm of the machine moved slowly and silently over my lower torso, the technician explained its millimeter-by-millimeter movement. I viewed its progress on the display terminal. As I watched, the five lower vertebrae of my spine appeared in color on the terminal. That completed, the technician repositioned me so the machine could study my hip. Later, the tests were analyzed, then compared to the first and only other test that I had had done, in 1987, the results of which had been excellent. My doctor happily informed me that I had not only maintained, but had actually built, bone in the past five years. May you have the same positive results!

54. WHAT IS THE DPA TEST?

Another procedure for measuring bone is DPA, which stands for Dual-Photon Absorptiometry, an older version of DEXA. This is a technique that measures the total bone-mineral content of the hip and spine. Using DPA, the patient is exposed to only slightly more radiation than a DEXA, but still less than than of a routine chest X-ray. It is a slower procedure and may be slightly less expensive than DEXA.

55. WHAT IS THE SPA TEST?

SPA stands for Single-Photon Absorptiometry. This test measures bone-mineral content mainly in the heel or wrist and forearm. The procedure measures cortical bone, which, although its loss can be a predictor of osteoporosis, does not predict nearly as well as the measurement of trabecular bone. (Cortical and trabecular bone are described on page 31, Question 4.) Sometimes SPA is used to measure the bone-mineral content of the heel, yet the accuracy of this measurement is debated.

A number of companies are currently seeking the approval of the Federal Drug Administration (FDA) for using heel measurement as a technique for testing for osteoporosis. Other experts believe that measurement of the heel is of questionable diagnostic value, because the heel bears so much weight that readings would be distorted.

You may wonder why traditional X-rays are not used to detect bone loss, inasmuch as we are familiar with their role in detecting bone breaks. They are not used because they are not sensitive enough to measure bone density and, thus, cannot pick up osteoporosis until 25 to 40 percent of bone loss has occurred, indicating that osteoporosis is well advanced.

56. WHAT IS AN RA TEST?

Radiographic Absorptiometry (RA) measures the bone-mineral content from X-rays of the hand, which are taken with a regular X-ray machine, then subjected to computer-controlled analysis.

57. WHAT IS COMPUTERIZED TOMOGRAPHY?

Computerized tomography, popularly referred to as CAT scan, can also measure bone density, but it exposes you to more radiation than the other procedures and can be more expensive. When it is used to measure spinal bone density, you may hear this procedure referred to as QCT, or Quantitative Computed Tomography. This procedure is unique in that it can measure the trabecular bone separately from the cortical bone.

58. WHAT EXACTLY DOES A BONE-DENSITY TEST SHOW?

Different bone-density tests use different measurements, but they all show essentially the same thing—the amount of mineral density in the bones. Your doctor may choose a particular test based on what site he or she is concerned about. For example, the QCT measures the density of a small amount of trabecular bone inside the vertebrae where, especially after menopause, changes may be the most rapid. DPA measures bone density independent of soft tissue in the lumbar spine, hip, or total body. DEXA is used for the hip, wrist, or spine and can measure the total calcium in the body. The RA looks at bone loss in appendages such as hands. Ultimately, if the test shows that your bone density is high, it means that you are at the lowest risk for osteoporosis.

59. YOU MENTIONED A NEW ULTRASOUND HEEL-SCREENING
    DEVICE. WOULD THAT ELIMINATE THE NEED FOR BONE
    DENSITOMETRY? IS IT EXPENSIVE?

The heel-screening device is purely experimental at
this writing. Applications for its use are pending approval
by the FDA. It does, however, appear to be a good
screening device because of the predictive nature of bone
loss in the heel, which can indicate bone loss in the spine
or elsewhere in the skeletal system. It is quick and painless
and can tell physicians which women need the more
expensive bone-density test. The heel device is based on
ultrasound waves, rather than X-ray. It works similarly to
sonar waves, which pass through water and bounce off
objects (such as submarines, when used by the military).
Although cost has not been determined, it is estimated
that the heel test will be far less expensive. However, some
experts question the value of this test because the heel
bears so much weight.

60. IS BONE-DENSITY TESTING DONE AS PART OF A ROUTINE
    EXAMINATION?

Not usually. Based on your risk factors for osteoporosis, your physician may decide that you need these tests to
determine whether you have lost bone, to decide whether
you should start on estrogen replacement therapy to
prevent bone loss, to monitor bone density if you're on

steroids or other medications that can affect bone density, or, if you have a vertebral deformity, whether you're suffering from osteoporosis. Some physicians routinely recommend a bone-density test around the time of menopause to get a baseline reading, wisely planning to retest you during the years of rapid bone loss that occurs during menopause to see if bone loss is accelerating beyond normal levels.

61. HOW EXPENSIVE IS A BONE-DENSITY TEST?

The cost of bone densitometry varies throughout the United States and depends on which procedure is performed. I have seen figures ranging from fifty dollars to two hundred and fifty dollars for these tests.

62. WILL MY MEDICAL INSURANCE COVER A BONE-DENSITY TEST?

At this writing, many insurance policies do not cover bone densitometry for diagnostic or screening purposes. This is probably because the U.S. health-care delivery system is set up to handle crisis care rather than preventive care, a situation that we all can work to modify. In the National Family Opinion Survey mentioned earlier, 83 percent of women surveyed felt that testing for osteoporosis in women over forty should be covered by medical insurance. Just as mammography for screening purposes finally is covered by most health insurance plans in many states and by the federally funded programs of Medicare and Medicaid, so we should encourage our insurers and our elected government officials to consider covering mass screening for osteoporosis.* Remember those 1.5 million fractures annually that we discussed on page 31? Well, in 1990 they cost us *ten billion* dollars in medical, social, and nursing-home costs, untold amounts of suffering and untimely deaths. If we don't stem the tide of this potential epidemic, it is projected that the cost will rise to sixty billion dollars in the next two or three decades.

* In the absence of a federal policy, ten states so far have adopted their own Medicare, Part B, reimbursement policies for bone-mass measurement.

63. WHERE CAN I GET A BONE-DENSITY TEST?

Bone densitometry is most often performed in the radiology departments of large hospitals and health-care facilities. Today, with the establishment of more menopause clinics, bone densitometry is coming into the clinic or office setting. If you are interested in having such a test, you need a referral from your physician as well as information on where such tests are available in your community.

64. HOW IMPORTANT IS IT FOR ME TO KNOW MY BONE
DENSITY, IF I'M ALREADY ALTERING MY DIET REGIMEN
AND EXERCISE PROGRAM?

That's a good question for your physician, who knows
your medical history (and family medical history) and has
examined you. Physicians tell me that many women quite
simply are not candidates for osteoporosis, based on their
lack of risk factors and their life-styles. Talk it over with
your doctor. You may be one of those women. (Yet,
according to the National Osteoporosis Foundation, un-
fortunately, some women with none of the risk factors do
develop osteoporosis.)

65. I'M FORTY-SIX YEARS OLD. I HAVE ALL THE RISK FACTORS
FOR OSTEOPOROSIS, EXCEPT THAT I DON'T SMOKE. I
WANT TO HAVE A BONE-DENSITY TEST PERFORMED
BEFORE I START A WEIGHT-LIFTING PROGRAM. MY
INTERNIST THINKS IT'S "UNNECESSARY," BECAUSE I'M
"STILL YOUNG." SHOULD I PUSH FOR A BONE-DENSITY
TEST NOW, OR NOT?

Here again, what's your relationship with your physician? Has he or she explained to you why the test is not
thought to be recommended for you? I think not, or you
would be more comfortable with the information. "Still
young" would not satisfy me as a reason, either. I suggest

that you ask your doctor to explain the medical reasons for that decision. The answer seems unsatisfactory, but your physician may have been thinking that a light weight-lifting program would strengthen your bones before you enter the rapid bone loss period that follows menopause. But, if you are still in doubt, ask directly to be referred for bone densitometry—most likely you'll be paying for it yourself, anyway. If that doesn't solve the problem, you probably should consider shopping around for a new doctor with whom you feel more satisfied. P.S. I'm glad you don't smoke!

66. BEFORE I CONSIDER TAKING ESTROGEN REPLACEMENT THERAPY, IS IT REASONABLE TO CHECK BONE DENSITY WITH AN INITIAL TEST, FOLLOWED BY REGULAR TESTING TO MONITOR BONE-DENSITY LOSS?

Doctors tell me that they refer a woman for bone densitometry when they are trying to make a decision about the appropriateness of estrogen replacement therapy as a preventive for osteoporosis or for the other reasons explained in the answer to Question 60. Frequently repeated bone-density testing seems excessive, not to mention expensive, if there is no disease present. Also, there are other reasons for considering ERT, so I think a candid and open discussion with your physician is called for.

Frankly, I was delighted to have a DEXA performed the first year I was in menopause. The results assured me that my bones were in good shape and that with effort on my part, I should be able to keep them strong during and after my menopausal years.

67. WHO SHOULD INTERPRET THE RESULTS OF THE BONE-DENSITY TEST?

That depends on which type of test is performed on you, but in most instances it will be read by a radiologist or by a physician specializing in osteoporosis.

68. SHOULD MEN HAVE BONE-DENSITY TESTING DONE, TOO?

Of the twenty-five million Americans who suffer from osteoporosis, five million are men. Most often, they are elderly men. Of the quarter-million senior adults who fracture their hips each year, more than one-fifth are men. Usually, men have Type II osteoporosis, also known as senile osteoporosis, which can affect both men and women, although it is not nearly as prevalent as postmenopausal osteoporosis, which is called Type I. Type II results from the slow bone loss related to the natural aging process in people over seventy years of age. Men are eligible for many of the same risk factors as women for getting the disease, such as a calcium-poor diet and sedentary life-style, and should not discount any of them with the exception of menopause. (Risk factors are discussed in Chapter Three.) Although male osteoporosis is not common, men with the risk factors for the disease may be referred for bone densitometry if the physician thinks the test is appropriate.

Osteoporosis occurs about ten years later in men than in women because men do not experience the hormonal changes and rapid bone loss that affect women in the seven-to-ten-year period after menopause. According to B. Lawrence Riggs, M.D., professor of medicine at the Mayo Clinic and past president of the National Osteoporosis Foundation, commenting in *USA Today*, "If it were not for menopause . . . the incidence of osteoporosis would probably be equal in men and women."

An important fact to remember is that bone densitometry is a diagnostic tool that is employed along with a full medical history and a complete physical examination and blood-chemistry testing to arrive at a diagnosis and treatment. It is important that both women and men learn in their younger years of the risk of osteoporosis in their later years, so that they can intervene successfully through life-style changes, coupled with the help of medical technology and treatment.

The strength of our democracy and our country is really no greater in the final analysis than the well-being of our citizens. The vigor of our country, its physical vigor and energy, is going to be no more advanced, no more substantial, than the vitality and will of our countrymen.

> President John F. Kennedy,
> July 19, 1961,
> remarks on Youth Fitness Program, quoted in
> Caroline Thomas Harnsberger,
> *Treasury of Presidential Quotations*
> (Follett Publishing, 1964).

CHAPTER 5

➤

How Can I Bone Up?

In the previous chapter, "boning up" was described as investigating, or studying, something that interests us. What could be more interesting than boning up on how to preserve and enhance our own good health and to prolong it over our long lives? How can we create and live a life-style that will at once please us and benefit us? We do it with careful thought and planning!

First we seek knowledge, and more and more women and men are doing just that by reading about the health issues (such as osteoporosis) surrounding menopause and midlife, and by educating themselves about what they can do to achieve a good-quality second half of adult life. Attendance of both women and men continues to grow at the programs in which I participate across the country, and they are asking pertinent questions at these programs.

Another interesting phenomenon that I've noticed: The average age of the women who attend the programs is dropping. Now, more than 75 percent of our audience is in the forty- to fifty-nine-year age range, with most attendees being premenopausal women aged forty to forty-nine. It's not that the number of postmenopausal women in attendance has dropped proportionately; it's that the size of the audience has grown!

Another most interesting finding is that beginning in 1992, more than one half of the women who completed our questionnaires correctly identified the risk factors for osteoporosis, noted that they were at risk, and indicated that they wanted to know more about this disease. (Fortunately, only a small percentage reported that they had already experienced osteoporosis.)

Three-fourths of the audiences correctly identified the following factors as being important in preventing osteoporosis, and placed them in this order of effectiveness: proper diet, exercise, calcium supplements, taking estrogen, and drinking milk.

I was delighted to learn that, following our program, a full 75 percent of women in our audiences indicated on their questionnaires that they now felt more confident about asking questions of their physicians (and they expected answers). Half said that they would visit their physicians soon; two-thirds stated that they would improve their daily diets and their exercise habits; and half noted that they would consider estrogen replacement therapy.

Women also offered additional changes that they were

planning to make: "keep closer contact with my doctor"; "take calcium supplements"; "be more relaxed"; "talk to my daughters and explain what's going on with me." Others wrote in these comments: "I'm premenopausal—I'm going to get on a weight-bearing exercise program—fast!"; "I'm at greater risk of osteoporosis than I thought"; "I learned that menopause and osteoporosis are connected"; "I learned not to take calcium with fiber"; "I'm learning to like skim milk"; "I learned that it's never too late to take measures to prevent osteoporosis or to stop it in its tracks"; "I learned the seriousness of osteoporosis"; "I think I might change doctors"; and "I know now that I've got to take charge of all of this myself."

A few sad notes were also offered. For example: "I have osteoporosis. I'm eighty-three and eight-and-a-half inches shorter than I used to be. I learned a lot this evening, but I wish someone had told me all this about forty years ago. Would you believe that when I was in my sixties, I cracked two ribs while I was just changing the sheets on the bed? Now, I'm extra careful with whatever I do or wherever I go and I'm trying not to break that hip that might do me in. So far, so good."

In 1992, on television in Cleveland, I heard Bernadine Healy, M.D., then the director of the National Institutes of Health (NIH), compare the annual cost of treating osteoporosis in the United States (ten billion dollars) to the entire annual budget of the NIH, also ten billion dollars. So you can see that the amount of money that is spent on osteoporosis research can only be a fraction of what it costs to treat this disease. If we don't do something about that, the balance will shift further as, with out projected longer life span, the U.S. population of older people increases. Better bone up!

The answers to the next ten questions that women asked at most of our programs should help you to do that.

69. ONCE BONE DENSITY HAS BEEN LOST, CAN IT BE REGAINED OR REPLACED?

It is said in some scientific circles that "bone lost is bone gone." Yet some interesting studies seem to ameliorate that fact somewhat. The most notable study was performed in a retirement community in southern California and is referred to as the Leisure World Study. In that study, a number of men and women over seventy who had not exercised in the past were put on a weight-bearing exercise program. Their bone density was measured before they began the program and again at its conclusion. The remarkable results indicated that some participants actually built bone mass during the exercise program, and this was true even for people in their eighties!

If you have suffered minor bone loss, it might be a good idea to discuss with your physician what you can do to try to rebuild bone, or at least to prevent further bone loss.

Among the life-style changes and therapies that might be considered are calcium supplementation, estrogen replacement therapy, and changes in your diet and exercise program. All of these are discussed in later chapters.

70. IS IT TRUE THAT CONSUMING TOO MUCH PROTEIN DECREASES BONE MASS BY STEALING THE CALCIUM FROM OUR BONES?

Yes. Excess protein can upset the body's pH balance, which leads to calcium loss. Here's how. Too much protein causes the body's pH to become too acidic. To correct this imbalance, calcium and phosphorus are leached from the bones to serve as a buffer for this acidic state. That drain of calcium causes our bones to weaken.

Anything that you do to throw the body's chemistry out of kilter, such as eating excessive amounts of protein, will have other effects as well. Some studies have shown that a diet high in protein creates a drop in your phosphorus level; that drop causes you to lose too much calcium through your urine—calcium that would have been working for you if it had maintained its balanced relationship to the phosphorus. Remember those all-protein or high-protein diets for quick weight loss that many of us went on? "Lose ten pounds in ten days," they proclaimed. Forget them!

So, you may be asking: How much protein should I eat? It's an individual matter. According to *The Mount Sinai*

School of Medicine Complete Book of Nutrition (St. Martin's Press, 1990), the amount of protein each of us needs depends on our age, body size, the composition of our diet, our state of health, and other factors. The daily recommendation for adults age nineteen and over is .036 gram of protein for each pound of ideal body weight. That means that if your ideal weight (not cosmetically, but for good health) is 150 pounds, you should consume about 50 grams of protein a day. (Americans, on average, consume twice that amount.) A talk with a dietitian or qualified nutritionist should bring a concrete answer for your particular physiology.

71. DO SOFT DRINKS BLOCK THE ABSORPTION OF CALCIUM INTO OUR BONES?

In the answer to the previous question, I explained that calcium and phosphorus work in harmony in our body chemistry: The ideal ratio is 2.5 parts calcium to 1 part phosphorus. All kinds of soft drinks—the sugar-free and caffeine-free varieties, as well as regular—contain phosphoric acid, which is a form of phosphorus. Too many sodas equal too much phosphorus, and that means an imbalance in that important relationship that enables our calcium to work for us. Instead of working to build bone, calcium is pulled out of our bones as the body tries to recreate the harmonious chemical balance that it requires.

So what can you do? Limit your sodas to one per day, if you can. According to Salt Lake City obstetrician/gynecologist Dr. Mary Beard, "... two at most."

72. I'VE HEARD THAT TOO MUCH CAFFEINE CAN KEEP US FROM ABSORBING CALCIUM. HOW DOES THAT HAPPEN?

Caffeine is a diuretic; that is, it is an agent that causes us to secrete more urine than we would otherwise. Our increased urine output is rich with minerals and, as we have seen in the answers to the first two questions in this chapter, that excessive loss of minerals from our bodies creates imbalances in our body chemistry. So, consuming too much caffeine will cause us to lose too much calcium, sodium, magnesium, and potassium in our urine. Now that you know that we need our calcium to protect our bones from osteoporosis, you can see how too much caffeine will deplete the body of calcium by causing us to excrete it.

Coffee is not the only place where we find caffeine. It is also in tea, chocolate, and soft drinks. It is wise to think about switching to decaffeinated coffees and teas. (I still have my two cups of "real" coffee in the morning, but I switch after that to decaf.) You may be surprised to learn how many prescription drugs and over-the-counter remedies for a wide assortment of common symptoms, such as medications for colds and coughs, contain caffeine. So read labels and talk to your pharmacist about the caffeine contained in various preparations.

How Can I Bone Up?

73. I DRINK VERY LITTLE MILK. HOW MANY MILLIGRAMS OF CALCIUM SHOULD I CONSUME EACH DAY?

The National Osteoporosis Foundation suggests that women consume 1,000 milligrams of calcium a day before menopause and 1,500 milligrams during and after menopause, if they are not taking estrogen (during and after menopause if a woman is taking estrogen, she can remain at 1,000 milligrams of calcium); that children and young women ages eleven through twenty-five, pregnant women, and nursing mothers take in 1,200 milligrams daily; and that children up to age ten take in 800 milligrams per day.

Dairy products are our richest sources of calcium. I find that with dairy products it is fairly easy to consume the amount of calcium one needs. For example, an eight-ounce glass of skim milk provides approximately 300 milligrams of calcium; certain nonfat yogurts provide another 350 milligrams per eight-ounce container (read the labels so that you can get the highest amount of calcium), and two calcium carbonate tablets (for example, Tums or Rolaids) provide another 400 or more milligrams. That's more than 1,000 milligrams daily. If we eat nutritious meals, we all consume approximately 400 more milligrams of calcium. If you don't like milk, consider yogurt, calcium-fortified orange juice, calcium-fortified cereals, beans, sardines and salmon with the bones in, and certain cheeses (if you're not watching your cholesterol), all of which can add significantly to fulfilling your daily calcium requirements. A diet rich in broccoli is also a good source of calcium as are other greens. Remember, though, that some green vegetables—asparagus, beet greens, Swiss chard, dandelion greens, parsley, rhubarb, and spinach—contain oxalates, which bind with calcium and block its absorption into your bones, so limit your consumption of those greens or use lemon to nullify oxalates.

While we're discussing calcium-rich foods, let's remember that children and adults up to the age of thirty-five are still working on building peak bone mass. Three eight-ounce servings of whole milk satisfy the requirements for our young children, and four servings of milk—whole, 2 percent, 1 percent, or skim—equal 1,200 milligrams of calcium—just the amount that teenagers and adults under thirty-five need.

74. AT WHAT AGE SHOULD I BEGIN TO COUNT CALCIUM MILLIGRAMS TO MAKE SURE THAT MY DAILY CALCIUM INTAKE WILL PROTECT MY BONES?

Ideally, that would occur in childhood, when you are building bone, and continue up through the teenage, young-adult, child-bearing, and premenopausal years, and into the postmenopausal years. But it's never too late to start. Look at the calcium Recommended Daily Allowance (RDA) for your age or stage of life (see Question 33) and begin counting now.

75. CAN YOU CONSUME TOO MUCH CALCIUM?

If you're asking, "If 1,000 milligrams is good, is 2,000 milligrams better?"—the answer is probably "no." Excessive amounts of calcium, whether taken by supplementation or food, can upset your body chemistry and can actually be harmful.

76. I'M SIXTY-TWO AND HAVE NEVER BROKEN A BONE IN MY LIFE. DOES THAT MEAN I HAVE A HIGH BONE DENSITY?

Not necessarily. It probably means that you have never had occasion to break a bone. I don't mean to sound glib, but there is no sure way to assess the silent thievery of osteoporosis except through a bone-density test. If you are seeking real reassurance, talk it over with your physician, and if your risk-factor analysis indicates that you are a candidate for osteoporosis, ask for a bone-density test.

77. I HAVE HAD SCOLIOSIS AND I HAVE A HISTORY OF CANCER IN MY FAMILY. THE CANCER MAKES ME AFRAID OF TAKING ESTROGEN. IS THERE ANYTHING ELSE THAT CAN PROTECT ME FROM BROKEN BONES?

The physicians with whom I discussed your question indicated that they are unaware, in most cases, of estrogen being contraindicated for women who have had scoliosis. Quite the reverse is true: Since people who have had scoliosis are at a higher risk for osteoporosis, estrogen may be beneficial. A family history of cancer may be another matter. Only your physician, who is aware of your medical and family history, can answer your question. If estrogen replacement therapy is not a consideration for you, either medically or because of your personal preference, why not discuss with your doctor how diet, exercise, and calcium supplementation or other medications to prevent bone loss, such as calcitonin, can protect your bones.

78. I HAVE TWO CHILDREN AND AM NOW PREGNANT WITH TWINS. DOES HAVING MANY CHILDREN DEPLETE BONE MASS, AND DOES HAVING MULTIPLE BIRTHS INCREASE THE DEPLETION?

Pregnancy can, indeed, deplete your bone mass, but only if you are not consuming enough calcium (about 1,200 milligrams are needed per day) to allow you to share calcium with your unborn babies. Without the extra calcium, your body will meet the infants' needs by taking calcium from your bones. I have found no studies indicating that multiple births require greater calcium consumption during pregnancy. Perhaps that is because, on average, multiple births deliver smaller individual babies, so that you may be sharing calcium with infants who, because of their size, together need only as much calcium as one baby.

How Can I Bone Up?

This chapter has explained the excesses to avoid in our diets and how we can ingest and keep our calcium so that we can protect the strength of our bones. The next few chapters deal with what we can do in terms of exercise, calcium supplementation, and hormone replacement in order to protect ourselves from osteoporosis. There are many things you can do to prevent one of the most crippling diseases of aging. Said much more simply:

The arrow seen before, cometh less rudely.

Dante, *The Divine Comedy* "Paradiso" 17

CHAPTER 6

What Kinds of Exercises Keep
Bones Strong?

A letter arrived the other day from a woman on the West Coast. She wrote:

I had to write to tell you that for a long time I have thought that each transition into a new stage of womanhood was designed to test me. From the moment I entered puberty and began to menstruate, I knew I was having a bad time.

My periods were never easy, and I think I always had PMS in a big way. Only back then, what I was having didn't even have the dignity of a name or an acronym. I just gave up two weeks of the month to feeling nervous and rotten . . . and to craving and overeating junk foods.

Finally, I began to hear that premenstrual tension was being treated as a "real" complaint, so I learned, at long last, that I wasn't "nuts" anymore. Once I had those initials— PMS—to support and encourage me, I found a physician who would listen and felt she could help me with my malady.

What Kinds of Exercises Keep Bones Strong?

Believe it or not, the activity that has helped me the most is exercise. I have actually been able to live through my menstrual cycle without driving my family and coworkers crazy.

I'm forty-four and just beginning to experience some of the symptoms of menopause and to learn about osteoporosis. Boy, am I exercising now!

Exercise, and what it can and should do for us, is a fairly complex subject, but one that is worth learning about. Exercise can be an inexpensive, nondrug mood and health enhancer that we can engage in with companions or alone, that we can keep up with no matter where we are, and, properly chosen, that we can do for the rest of our lives. Yet, according to Barbara Drinkwater, Ph.D., speaking at a meeting of the North American Menopause Society in Cleveland in September 1992, "Only one-third of physicians discuss exercise with their patients, and less than 10 percent of the population exercises on a regular basis."

Recently, I heard osteoporosis intervention described as a "three-legged stool." One leg is nutrition, the second is exercise, and the third is estrogen replacement therapy. *Exercise is the only way, known today, to build bone density after we've stopped growing.* We can build it by stressing the bone. How does that work? Let's look at the tennis professional's favored arm. It's somewhat larger than the less-used arm, and studies have shown that that difference is found in both the muscle and the bone.

There is no definitive reason that explains why this occurs. According to the National Osteoporosis Foundation's *Physician's Resource Manual on Osteoporosis* (1991), "Mechanical forces are known to promote bone growth, and exposure of bones to such forces can enhance bone density. . . . Why physical activity influences bone density is unclear, although {we do know that} mechanical forces promote osteoblast growth and activity." Weight-bearing exercise provides that mechanical force.

Clearly, exercise is vital to us at all ages. I have a new friend (I'll call her Alice) whom I met at a spa in 1992, where I was presenting a program on menopause. Alice was distraught, because when she was measured quickly upon her arrival, she was told that she had lost three-quarters of an inch in height. "I won't get hysterical," she said, "until I've been measured again when I get home." I thought that was reasonable and couldn't account for her heightened distress until she said, "I'm forty-seven, and I've had osteoporosis for at least fifteen years! When I was thirty-seven, the doctor told me I had the bones of a sixty-year-old woman. I wonder how bad they are now." (Alice had just returned from two years in the Far East and hadn't been seen by her physician since her return.) She asked me to share her story with my readers.

When she was fourteen, Alice had one-and-a-half ovaries removed because of a football-size benign cyst on her right ovary. This was a fluid-filled cyst (which accounted for its size) that could have ruptured at any time. She told me:

> I must have had it for a while before it was found, because the family doctor to whom my mother took me was reluctant to do an internal examination on an adolescent. He told my mom that I was probably just bloated because I was going through puberty.
>
> I remember what I looked like. There I was, a skinny little thing with this great big abdomen. I was even embarrassed to get undressed for gym class. Finally, my mother realized something was really wrong and took me to her gynecologist. . . . When he removed the cyst, he had to take out the right ovary and part of the left, but he tried to save one piece of ovary for me.
>
> I was never told of this. I never knew that they had taken more than half of the other ovary out. My mother never told me, because she didn't want me to worry. She told me later that she just prayed I wouldn't wait too long to have children. I was lucky. I got married at twenty and got pregnant easily with my first child when I was twenty-three and with my second a year and a half later. Then I learned how little ovary I actually had left.
>
> Then my periods started to get irregular. At my annual gynecology examination when I was thirty-two, the doctor found another cyst on my remaining piece of ovary. The

ovary was removed, as was my uterus, in a hysterectomy, probably because he believed my uterus no longer served any worthwhile purpose. I was put on estrogen therapy. When I was thirty-seven, I learned I had osteoporosis. It actually had shown up on the routine chest X-ray I'd had prior to the hysterectomy five years earlier, but no one had said anything about it. Then came high doses of calcium, but the only exercise I was doing was swimming and I didn't know that swimming wouldn't do much for my bones. {More about that later in this chapter.} Two years later, I had another bone densitometry test, and I had lost more bone.

Then I began weight-bearing exercises in earnest, and I was trying to eat as much calcium-rich food as I could handle. When I was forty-five and went back to the clinic, I learned that my bone loss had stopped. I hadn't gained bone, but my new regimen was stemming the loss. I'm going in for my next bone-density test soon. Wish me luck. I'll call and let you know how I'm doing.

I'm happy to report that the spa measurement was in error (Alice thinks that maybe she wasn't standing up tall), and that Alice is still hanging on to the bone mass last reported. She's still watching her diet and doing weight-bearing exercises in a regular planned program. Alice is hopeful that she can prevent further bone loss.

79. HOW IS NEW BONE MADE, AND HOW DOES WEIGHT-BEARING EXERCISE HELP BONES?

What Kinds of Exercises Keep Bones Strong?

Researchers now know that new cortical bone is laid down in concentric circles; these are actually called Haversian canals. Bone is also increased at trabecular sites when the holes left by the resorption process are refilled. Weight-bearing exercise thickens bone by increasing blood flow within those canals. The increased blood brings with it extra nutrients for the bone-building cells. Weight-bearing exercise also puts stress on the bones—creating an electrical charge within the Haversian canals that stimulates the bone-building cells.

80. I'M HEALTHY. WHY DO I NEED TO EXERCISE SO OFTEN?

As we know, exercise can play a role in either preventing or ameliorating many diseases, including high blood pressure, diabetes, heart disease, stroke, and arthritis, as well as osteoporosis. Exercise also can help us fight depression, constipation, insomnia, and weight gain. Its benefits are invaluable. However, before you start an exercise program that is new for you, check with your physician.

81. HOW DO I FIGURE OUT WHAT KINDS OF EXERCISES I SHOULD DO?

To create the ideal exercise program for our bones, our hearts, and the rest of our bodies, we need to incorporate three kinds of exercise: stretching for flexibility; aerobic exercises for heart and lungs; and weight-bearing exercises for bones. Ideally, the right amount of each form of exercise should be worked out for us on an individual basis. For many of us, that is not possible, so this chapter will contain information about how to design your own program.

The goals of an exercise program might include making us feel like healthy, strong, active women; maintaining our bone mass; increasing our lean muscle mass and reducing the fat in our bodies; enabling us to do more with less fatigue; and fulfilling our desire to remain active and independent until the end of our lives.

82. I START EXERCISING WITH ENTHUSIASM AND STOP BECAUSE I'M SO BUSY. HOW CAN I FIND THE TIME FOR ALL THIS EXERCISE?

Exercise should be a lifetime commitment for the maintenance of our good health, which must include maintaining our bone mass. If you stop exercising, you can quickly lose what you've gained. Studies show, and athletes agree, that detraining occurs very quickly. So then, how come so few of us exercise regularly? Many women who talk to me after the programs tell me that they just don't have time to exercise. I find myself explaining frequently that I don't perform my entire exercise program every day, but that I alternate activities. And when my travel schedule or hotel accommodations offer no way to exercise, I simply walk whenever and wherever I can. Remember that you can divide your exercise program up into shorter sessions, if you don't have an hour to spare.

If I could make clear how much easier and more time efficient it is to stay active and healthy, maintain bone mass, and possibly prevent fractures than it is to try to fix what's been broken, my goal will have been reached. If you exercise and maintain bone mass, aerobic capacity, and flexibility, you will reach yours.

83. WHAT KIND OF EXERCISE PROGRAM WILL FULFILL ALL MY BODY'S NEEDS?

The guidelines of the American College of Sports Medicine (ACSM) call for us to perform three aerobic and two strength-training workouts each week. Each workout should be preceded and followed by a five-to-ten minute stretching session.

In its plan for exercise-testing and prescription, the ACSM divides exercise into two categories—moderate and vigorous. They are quite different for each individual, depending on the health status and the exercise goals of the person. By ACSM's definition, moderate means that you are exercising at 40 to 60 percent of your capacity, or target heart rate, for sixty minutes. In a vigorous program you would work at more than 60 percent of your capacity for fifteen to twenty minutes. This is true for aerobic exercise, in which your body's oxygen demand should equal its oxygen supply.

84. How do I figure out my target heart rate?

Aerobic exercise uses large-muscle mass continuously at our target heart rate. To determine that, subtract your age from 220, then calculate 70 to 80 percent of that figure. (For example, if you are fifty, 220 minus 50 equals 170. Now multiply 170 × .70 {119} and 170 × .80 {136}. Your target heart rate is between 119 and 136 beats per minute.) Ideally, you should do your aerobic exercise three to four times a week for forty-five to sixty minutes each time. (This will also help burn fat.) You also can split one day's exercise into two separate thirty-minute segments. The idea here is that if you exercise at a lower capacity, you exercise longer. Aerobic exercise has positive implications for many diseases, as well as for our general good health and sense of well-being. The minimum amount of aerobic exercise that will protect us cardiovascularly is twenty to thirty minutes of aerobic exercise, three times a week.

85. What will weight lifting do for my bones?

What Kinds of Exercises Keep Bones Strong?

Today, exercise physiologists believe weight lifting (resistance training) to be one of the most effective exercise regimens for osteoporosis prevention. That is because lifting weights stresses your muscles which build mass, which in turn, puts stress on your bones, which can help to maintain, or even enhance, your bone density. Ideally, weight lifting two to three times per week with free weights or weight machines (such as Nautilus) and engaging in six to twelve repetitions of each lift at 60 to 80 percent of maximal strength will improve muscle strength and muscle endurance, and protect bones.

86. WHAT EXACTLY ARE WEIGHT-BEARING EXERCISES?

These are exercises in which you put stress on the bone. According to the National Osteoporosis Foundation, the following are the preferred weight-bearing exercises:

- Walking
- Stair Climbing
- Hiking
- Dancing
- Weight Training (free weights or weight machines)
- Jogging
- Skiing (downhill and cross-country)
- Aerobic Dance (low-impact)
- Treadmill

The next tier of suitable weight-bearing exercises is comprised of activities that are of lower impact:

- Cross-country ski machines
- Stair-climbing machines
- Stair-step machines
- Water aerobics

87. IS SWIMMING GOOD EXERCISE FOR ME AT THE MENOPAUSAL TIME OF LIFE?

Swimming is not classified as a weight-bearing exercise, so it would not enhance maintenance of bone mass. It does, however, offer flexibility training and some cardiovascular benefit. Perhaps swimming could be alternated with another weight-bearing exercise for maximum protection for your bones. Water aerobics and water-walking or water-jogging, however, are low-impact weight-bearing exercises.

88. I AM UNABLE TO DO ANY OF THE WEIGHT-BEARING EXERCISES BECAUSE I HAVE MULTIPLE SCLEROSIS. IS THERE ANY WATER EXERCISE THAT CAN HELP ME PROTECT MY BONES?

What Kinds of Exercises Keep Bones Strong?

Yes, try gentle water-aerobics classes or water walking. Women indicate that the buoyancy of the water helps with balance, and the resistance of the water adds weight-bearing qualities to these activities.

89. WHAT ABOUT LIFTING WEIGHTS? AND CAN'T THAT BE DANGEROUS FOR SOMEONE IN HER SIXTIES?

Whatever your age, before you begin any weight-lifting program, discuss it with your physician. There are several kinds of programs: Some women prefer machines, such as Nautilus or Universal; others like to use free weights; still others like to use wrist or ankle weights. And many women use some combination of the above. If you are in good health and if you begin slowly, with light weights and under the supervision of an exercise physiologist or a certified trainer, weight lifting can be a very positive and pleasing way to maintain bone.

Moreover, age seems to be no barrier to obtaining results. A 1990 study coauthored by William Evans, director of the physiology laboratory at the Human Nutrition Research Center on Aging at Tufts University, and reported in *The New York Times Magazine* (April 1991) indicated that "nine men and women between the ages of 87 and 96 increased the strength in the front of their thigh muscles by an average of 175 percent after eight weeks of supervised weight lifting."

90. I'M TWENTY-THREE. WHAT KIND OF AN EXERCISE PROGRAM SHOULD I BEGIN NOW TO PROTECT ME IN THE FUTURE?

Ideally, an exercise program should incorporate stretching for flexibility, aerobic activity for cardiovascular health, and weight-bearing exercise for enhancing bone mass. At your age, it is likely that you may still be building bone. What a good time to work toward enhancing peak bone mass, which we usually achieve around age thirty-five! Remember, we all lose bone mass at the rate of around 1 percent per year as we age. Obviously, having a higher peak mass from which to lose would be to your benefit.

91. WOULDN'T AN INCREASE IN MY AEROBIC EXERCISE PROGRAM HELP ME TO PREVENT OSTEOPOROSIS?

It would, because it is considered a preferred weight-bearing exercise. You might also want to consider adding resistance training, or weight training, two times a week, which is what the American College of Sports Medicine Guidelines suggest. So if you have more time, and you're in good health, why not consider adding weight lifting to your program, if your doctor agrees.

92. WHAT SHOULD A STRENGTH-TRAINING PROGRAM INCLUDE?

A balanced strength-training program should be designed to strengthen all of your major muscle groups—arms, shoulders, chest, back, abdomen, hips, and legs. If you can perform weight lifting twice each week, it's a good idea to balance those days in between your other exercise activities. For example, lift on Mondays and Thursdays or Wednesdays and Saturdays rather than two days in a row. Your muscles need time to recover.

93. HOW MANY CALORIES DOES WEIGHT LIFTING BURN?

Twenty to thirty minutes of weight lifting will usually burn between 200 and 300 calories, depending on your muscle mass and effort. More important, however, is that you will add muscle mass, and every pound of muscle that you build burns an extra 30 to 50 calories a day. Not bad!

94. WHY DOES EXERCISE CAUSE BONE LOSS IN YOUNG WOMEN AND PROTECT AGAINST BONE LOSS IN OLDER WOMEN?

Good question! But, let's look at this question carefully, because we're talking about matters of degree. Young women who exercise to an extent that does not in any way alter their hormonal balance or menstrual cycle are usually affecting their bones in a positive manner. It is only the young women who exercise so excessively that their periods stop, who are cautioned about the dangers of amenorrhea, which is caused by estrogen deficiency, and subsequent bone loss.

Postmenopausal women—in fact, all women—are encouraged to exercise appropriately to protect their bones in order to prevent osteoporosis, to promote cardiovascular health, and to encourage flexibility and strength.

95. I'VE HEARD SO MUCH ABOUT THE SAFETY AND ADVANTAGES OF A WALKING PROGRAM FOR EVERY AGE. CAN YOU TELL ME HOW MANY DAYS A WEEK I SHOULD PLAN TO WALK? HOW FAST AND FOR HOW LONG?

Walking is truly wonderful. Not sauntering, but walking a nice even deliberate pace. Three days a week of walking will usually meet your aerobic needs, but four or five would even be better. A good pace might be between a twenty- and a fifteen-minute mile. That would provide you with a three-to-four-mile walk an hour. Whatever your pace, you should still be able to hold a conversation comfortably.

In terms of the joys of walking, they include enabling us to enjoy nature if we're outside, to catch up on the latest news with a friend while doing something positive for our health, to broaden our friendships by joining a walking group or club, or to socialize while walking at a mall and then being in place to do our shopping. Many malls across the country are opening their doors early so that citizens of all ages can walk in comfort and safety.

There are other ways to cram in your walking program. Bypass the elevators in buildings and walk up the escalators or the stairs instead. Park your car in the spot in the parking lot farthest away from where you're going, and get in a walk going to and from the car. Or leave your car home altogether and walk to work, to shop, or to a friend's home if the distance and safety considerations make that feasible. Add some hilly areas to your outdoor walking program. Make arrangements to meet a friend outside for a walk, and don't be a "no-show." If we all could change the habit of conversing with a friend for a long time on the phone to walking and talking with that friend, both parties would benefit. With the addition of your Walkman, walking and listening to music or to a good book can be beneficial, too.

The problem with an exercise program is our own compliance with it. Yet studies have shown that women who have had their bone density tested and found it low, comply better with their exercise routine. Although no long-term studies have yet *fully* shown how wonderfully beneficial exercise might be to us as we age, researchers today know that one of the ways that we can preserve our bone mass is with exercise, and that the lower our bone density, the greater our risk of bone fractures.

An interesting note was struck at the North American Menopause Meeting, September 1992, by Morris Notelovitz, M.D., a leader in the field of menopause, osteoporosis, and women's health. Dr. Notelovitz noted that although Japanese women have lower bone density than white American women, they sustain fewer fractures. He postulated that perhaps that is because the squat is a resting position for them and they frequently are seen comfortably squatting even while waiting for a bus, thus stressing their muscles and strengthening their bones. Walking is easier!

There is so much beauty out of doors that so many of us miss as we go about the busyness of our lives. I cannot encourage you enough to go outdoors for a long walk and drink in the sights and sounds of each season. They go by so quickly! Try not to miss a single day.

Recently, in a small volume, a quote by a ballerina extraordinaire caught my eye and imagination:

Life forms illogical patterns. It is haphazard and full of beauties which I try to catch as they fly by, for who knows if any of them will ever return?

Margot Fonteyn, in
The Quotable Woman
(Running Press, 1992).

CHAPTER 7

What Kinds of Foods and Calcium Supplements Can Help Protect Bones?

A chilling article sent over Maturity News Service and reported in the Cleveland *Plain Dealer* (November 10, 1992) announced that the American Academy of Orthopedic Surgeons is "engineering a national prevention effort" to stem the tide of a hip-fracture "epidemic." These medical specialists were "launching a preemptive strike on the bone-thinning disease known as osteoporosis to head off a threatened epidemic of hip fractures that would overwhelm the health-care delivery system." The numbers bear out that warning!

More than a quarter-million Americans fracture their hips each year. Most of them are women over age sixty-five. As women, we have a 20 percent chance of breaking a hip at some time in our lives. These incredible numbers are not static. As the population of older women grows, the number of hip fractures will grow as well. The orthopedic surgeons' warning is rife with meaning!

It isn't as if these fractures mend easily or comfortably. The cost in pain and dollars is enormous. The cost in loss of independence seems even greater to me—even more than the estimated cost of thirty-five thousand dollars per patient to fix a hip fracture. Imagine—one out of two people who suffer hip fractures will *never* walk again! And from 12 to 20 percent of these will die within six months of their fractures, often from complications of surgery or from infection picked up afterward. In the aggregate, we're speaking of a total of ten billion health-care dollars annually, spent on osteoporosis alone!

This isn't how any of us wants to spend our "golden years." So what else can we do to protect outselves? We've already underscored the bone-enhancing importance of weight-bearing exercise in Chapter Six. In this chapter we're going to discuss further another important aspect touched on earlier for maintaining healthy bones: dietary and supplemental calcium. Later, in Chapter Eight, we'll assess the benefits of estrogen therapy, and in Chapter Nine, we'll review what other medications are available to treat osteoporosis.

Let's review how much calcium we need daily: 1,000 milligrams as premenopausal women and 1,500 milligrams at menopause and beyond. If we take estrogen and are not at high risk for osteoporosis, some studies show that we can stay at the 1,000-milligram level. Personally, although I have used the estrogen patch for several years and I do not fit the high-risk profile described in Chapter One, I still try to keep my daily calcium intake above the 1,000 milligram mark— closer to 1,200.

What Kinds of Foods Can Protect Bones?

An important report in the *Journal of the American Medical Association* (November 1992) announced that researchers have *definitively* established that women add bone mass long after adolescence and probably until they reach age thirty. The findings of this important study offer young women concrete knowledge that with moderate exercise and adequate calcium intake, they can avoid the ravages to their bones from osteoporosis when they age.

According to the chief author of the study, Robert B. Recker, M.D., professor of medicine at Creighton University Medical School in Omaha, this study clearly indicates that modest changes in life-style "can help to increase bone mass in young women age twenty to thirty." The study showed the importance of exercise, but it also revealed that the intake of calcium had the strongest effect on bone growth. Young women—my daughters and your daughters—take heed!

Writing in the November/December issue of *Menopause Management*, Myron Winick, M.D., emeritus professor of nutrition, Columbia University College of Physicians and Surgeons, explains that "when osteoporosis prevention is the goal, the most essential nutritional requirement is adequate dietary intake of the vital threshold nutrient, calcium."

96. HOW, THEN, DO WE DEFINE CALCIUM?

Calcium is a mineral nutrient that helps us build healthy bones and teeth. Yet in our bodies it behaves in a somewhat capricious manner. Our bones are unable to hold on to the calcium they need if we do not take in enough calcium in our diet for other needs. If our calcium intake is below our needs, our bodies right that imbalance by drawing calcium from the stores in our bones. For our good skeletal health, it is imperative that we get our calcium from the grocery stores and the pharmacy rather than from the stores in our bones.

Remember, too, that we lose calcium in our urine: between 150 and 200 milligrams per day. Information from the National Osteoporosis Foundation reveals that we consume far less calcium than we need. According to *Osteoporosis*, a booklet of the National Institutes of Health published in 1989 by the U.S. Department of Health and Human Services, the average calcium intake of the majority of middle-aged and elderly women falls somewhere between 450 and 550 milligrams per day. It doesn't take a mathematical whiz to see the problem here. Depending on our age, most of us short-change ourselves of 500 to 1,000 milligrams of calcium per day.

In studying the questionnaires I have gathered from the consumer programs, I can see that the number of women who understand the value of calcium intake is growing. More than half of the completed questionnaires from programs held during the fall of 1992 showed that learning about osteoporosis was women's number-one reason for attending. When asked about what actions were important in preventing osteoporosis, two-thirds of the women noted proper diet, exercise, taking estrogen and calcium supplements, and drinking milk (in that order of importance) as effective. Their answers were right on target, although drinking milk should be included with diet. The women cite being Caucasian or Asian as their number-one risk factor for osteoporosis; inadequate exercise as number two; and low calcium intake as number three.

The order in which the women identified these risk factors is borne out in the National Family Opinion Survey as well. From both the survey and the questionnaires, it is apparent, however, that many women do not know some of the other factors that can adversely affect their calcium balance, such as what prescriptions or over-the-counter drugs they may be taking or, to a lesser degree, the amount of caffeine or soda they consume.

In posing their questions at the programs, it is apparent that women want to close the information gap.

97. HOW MUCH CALCIUM SHOULD A WOMAN TAKE DAILY? DOES IT CHANGE WITH AGE?

As previously noted, a woman should take in 1,000 to 1,500 milligrams of calcium each day. Yes, the amount does change with age and also depends on your stage of life.

Our bodies cannot absorb or use calcium in the absence of vitamin D, the "sunshine vitamin." Please refer to Chapter Five, Questions 70 through 75, for additional information about calcium consumption and to Question 112 in this chapter for more about vitamin D.

98. WHAT FOODS, BESIDES MILK, CONTAIN CALCIUM?

Many women really have never thought about how to find calcium in foods other than dairy products. That's understandable, because dairy foods are deservedly known as the first-choice sources of dietary calcium. When we are born, milk is our first food! Without calcium intake from dairy products, your daily food consumption is drastically short of calcium. If the reason why you avoid dairy products has to do with watching dietary fat and cholesterol, solving the calcium problem is fairly simple. Just switch to skim milk and nonfat dairy products. Skim milk actually has about 11 more milligrams of calcium in each cup than whole milk does anyway, and it contains fewer calories than whole milk. To help you figure out how to get your daily calcium, I have included a chart from the National Osteoporosis Foundation that shows where to find calcium in foods.

SELECTED CALCIUM-RICH FOODS

FOOD ITEM	SERVING SIZE	CALCIUM (MG)	CALORIES
Milk			
Whole	8 oz.	291	150
Skim	8 oz.	302	85
Yogurt (with added milk solids)			
Plain, lowfat	8 oz.	415	145
Fruit, lowfat	8 oz.	343	230
Cheese			
Mozzarella, part skim	1 oz.	207	80
Muenster	1 oz.	203	105
Cheddar	1 oz.	204	115
Ricotta, part skim	4 oz.	335	190
Cottage, lowfat (2%)	4 oz.	78	103
Ice Cream, Vanilla (11% fat)			
Hard	1 cup	176	270
Soft serve	1 cup	236	375
Ice Milk, Vanilla			
Hard (4% fat)	1 cup	176	185
Soft serve (3% fat)	1 cup	274	225
Fish and Shellfish			
Sardines, canned in oil, drained, *including bones*	3 oz.	372	175
Salmon, pink, canned, *including bones*	3 oz.	167	120
Shrimp, canned, drained	3 oz.	98	100
Vegetables			
Bok Choy, raw	1 cup	74	9
Broccoli, cooked, drained, from raw	1 cup	136	40
Broccoli, cooked, drained, from frozen	1 cup	100	50
Soybeans, cooked, drained, from raw	1 cup	131	235
Collards, cooked, drained, from raw	1 cup	357	65
Turnip greens, cooked, drained, from raw (leaves and stems)	1 cup	252	30
Tofu	4 oz.	*108	85
Almonds	1 oz.	75	165

* The calcium content of tofu may vary depending on processing methods. Tofu processed with calcium salts can have as much as 300 mg calcium per 4 oz. Often, the label or the manufacturer can provide more specific information.

Used with permission of the *National Osteoporosis Foundation*.

99. IF I NEED CALCIUM, BUT CANNOT CONSUME (OR DIS-
    LIKE) DAIRY PRODUCTS, WILL CALCIUM SUPPLEMENTS
    WORK JUST AS WELL TO PROTECT ME FROM OSTEO-
    POROSIS?

Yes, but it would be best if you worked this out with
your own physician, or a dietitian or nutritionist. If you
want to try first to do it yourself, let's review the numbers.
As we've discussed earlier, the amount of calcium you need
depends on the age and stage of your life. Write down that
number. Can you figure out how much calcium you are
getting from other foods in your diet from our calcium-rich
food list on page 129? Subtract that amount from your
daily requirement. (The amount of calcium ingested from
the foods on the list is usually only about 450 milligrams
per day.) The number you have left is how much calcium
you still need to acquire through foods or supplementation.
First look to some food products that you might consider
including in your daily diet, such as calcium-fortified cereal
or calcium-fortified orange juice, which really do add
calcium to our diets. Subtract again. That is the number of
milligrams of calcium you need to obtain from calcium
supplements, providing you are not using drugs that leach
calcium from the bones, or drugs that stop, or limit,
calcium absorption; and provided you are not eating large
amounts of foods that inhibit calcium absorption, which
will be described later in this chapter. Now you have your

missing number. Take it to your pharmacist and get some help selecting the calcium supplement that is best for you. Remember to look for the word *elemental* on the package—that's the number of milligrams of pure calcium in the product. That's the actual amount of calcium you will receive. Calcium carbonate, often found in antacid products, can provide 200 milligrams of elemental calcium per 500-milligram tablet, and the highest amount of elemental calcium is usually found in calcium carbonates. (Do not try to get your calcium from bone meal or dolomite, as they may contain lead or other toxic metals.) Figure out how many tablets bring you even with your calcium need for your age. Then, before you begin, check your plan out with your doctor.

100. I'VE READ THAT SOME CALCIUM TABLETS ARE NOT EFFECTIVE, BECAUSE THEY DON'T DISSOLVE PROPERLY. WHAT ARE SOME GOOD CALCIUM TABLETS?

I've heard that, too. I recently learned that if you drop the calcium tablet that you are currently taking into half a glass of vinegar, stir, and it doesn't dissolve in thirty minutes—it's not disintegrating properly in your digestive tract, either. Physicians with whom I discussed this important question suggest that although calcium carbonates are generally the best sources of elemental calcium for us, supplements that combine calcium carbonate and calcium citrate may do the best job, because they do dissolve more readily and are less irritating to your digestive tract. Some names that appear high on their lists include Os-Cal and Caltrate. As for me, I stick with two Tums at bedtime. I take them at night because in that way, I have spaced my calcium consumption out over the course of each day, having had some calcium-rich foods at each meal. There seem to be differing schools of thought on when it is best to take your calcium supplements; some say it's best to take them with food because food stimulates the acid secretions in your stomach that are necessary to dissolve the calcium; others say it's best to take them at bedtime when they have all night to be absorbed into your digestive tract. Besides, at night we lose the most calcium because we are immobile and that could be a signal for our bodies to replace some of the lost calcium by drawing it from our bones.

101. WHAT EFFECT DOES ALCOHOL CONSUMPTION HAVE ON CALCIUM?

Excessive use, or abuse, of alcohol may contribute to osteoporosis because excessive alcohol consumption can be linked with poor eating habits, or because alcohol hinders the calcium absorption in the intestinal tract. Moderate alcohol use, such as one drink per day, does not seem to inhibit calcium absorption to any significant degree. That one drink may be one and one half ounces of scotch or bourbon (or your choice), six ounces of wine, or twelve ounces of beer.

102. WHAT FOODS ARE KNOWN TO BLOCK CALCIUM ABSORPTION?

Foods that contain compounds known as phytates or oxalates may inhibit calcium absorption. Phytates may be found in some whole-grain cereals, particularly those that use the outer husks of oatmeal and bran grains and in some legumes. Oxalate-containing foods include beets and beet greens, cocoa, dandelion greens, parsley, peanuts, rhubarb, spinach, summer squash, and tea. These are substances that should be eaten in moderation so as not to waste the calcium you have taken in from other foods.

103. WHAT KIND OF CALCIUM ABSORBS BEST?

Calcium carbonate is the form of calcium that is reported to be the best absorbed (sometimes combined with calcium citrate). Women seem to continue taking these preparations because with fewer tablets they can get the recommended amount of calcium, and because calcium carbonate contains the highest percentage of elemental calcium.

104. WHY DO PHYSICIANS SUGGEST AVOIDING TAKING FIBER AND CALCIUM-RICH FOODS TOGETHER? FOR EXAMPLE, WHAT ABOUT CEREAL AND MILK?

Let's think about the purpose of fiber, which is to move through and cleanse our systems and help with speedy, comfortable, and regular elimination. Calcium-rich foods—particularly dairy products—work best when they move slowly through our digestive tract, so that we can absorb their nutrients though our intestines. You can see how fiber, binding with the calcium in our intestines and moving it quickly through our digestive system, can defeat the calcium-absorption process and rob us of some of the calcium. It would be good to eat these nutrients separately, or in the case of cereal and milk, not to count the full value of the calcium consumed from the milk. I am unable to tell you officially how much of the calcium value you can count on; I just figure about half.

105. DOES CALCIUM SUPPLEMENTATION INTERFERE WITH THE IRON IN MY BODY?

A small study from Tufts University shows that in women who took extra calcium—up to 500 milligrams of elemental calcium with their meals—their ability to retain iron was decreased by more than 40 percent. Iron deficiency is a common problem for women, so it would seem appropriate to take calcium supplements separately from meals (but perhaps with a snack) in order to enable our bodies to absorb the iron that we need. It probably is best that women not take an iron pill or a vitamin with iron with their calcium pills.

Fifty-six percent of the women completing the questionnaires at our programs complained of fatigue. Fatigue may be a symptom of iron deficiency. It is a good idea to have your iron levels checked by your doctor, if fatigue is a problem for you. My semi-annual gynecological check-up has, for the past few years, included a simple finger-stick blood test to check my iron levels. However, whether or not you are taking calcium supplementation, I caution you not to self-dose with extra iron, since iron can be toxic and difficult to eliminate from your system. While you are having your iron levels checked, you might ask your doctor how to take your calcium supplement so that it does not interfere with iron absorption.

Recently, some research studies have looked to the possibility of a connection between excessive amounts of iron in the blood and heart disease. One of the working asumptions in this research endeavor is that women may begin to suffer coronary vascular disease (CVD) after menopause because of a build-up of iron in the blood. This iron formerly was expelled as part of the menstruation process. Although still in its very early stages, this hypothesis is being investigated, and the research reports emanating from it may be very interesting to health-conscious women.

106. SINCE MAGNESIUM ALSO AFFECTS BONE FORMATION, SHOULD I TAKE MAGNESIUM WITH MY CALCIUM SUPPLEMENTS?

If you drink milk, eat leafy green vegetables, seafood, dried beans, whole grains, and nuts, you are probably getting all the magnesium you need. If not, a good daily multivitamin usually includes enough magnesium. Remember, it is important to keep all our nutrients in balance.

107. IS IT POSSIBLE TO TAKE TOO MUCH CALCIUM?

Kidney stones may result from excessive amounts of calcium. Unless you already have a personal medical history of kidney stones, the recommended amounts of calcium do not constitute that threat. If, however, you have had kidney stones in the past, be sure to discuss with your doctor the amount of calcium you should ingest. Physicians usually do not recommend calcium supplements for people with kidney stones. The rule of thumb is that taking more calcium than you need does you no good, and amounts doubling your needs can indeed be harmful.

108. I CANNOT TOLERATE DAIRY PRODUCTS AND I DON'T WANT TO TAKE CALCIUM SUPPLEMENTS. CAN I CON-

What Kinds of Foods Can Protect Bones?

SUME ENOUGH CALCIUM TO PROTECT MY BONES
THROUGH DIET ALONE?

Yes, if you take the time to plan very carefully.
Actually, the best source of calcium is food. The National
Osteoporosis Foundation chart of calcium-rich foods can
be found on page 129. Use it to count milligrams of
calcium. However, if what you refer to is lactose intolerance (the inability to digest dairy products or an allergy to
them), perhaps you can still get some of your calcium from
yogurt (with active acidophilus cultures, which break
down the lactose, making yogurt easier to tolerate), hard
cheeses (if cholesterol is not a problem), and special milks,
such as Lactaid or Dairy Ease, that contain lactase, the
enzyme that digests milk sugars. There are also over-the-
counter preparations that contain lactase that may enable
you to consume dairy foods. Check them out with your
pharmacist. For some tips on packing calcium into your
daily menus, see Seven Ways in Seven Days to Pack
Calcium into Your Diet, at the end of this chapter.

109. DOES SALT INTAKE DIMINISH CALCIUM ABSORPTION?

A small amount of salt, or sodium, is naturally found
in our bones. It is one of the elements that helps to hold
our calcium and phosphorus together. However, if too
much salt is consumed, we risk losing some calcium from
our bones. It is thought to occur this way: The more

sodium we consume, the more sodium we excrete and the more calcium goes out with it. The calcium that we lose in this fashion does not come from the amount absorbed through our digestive tract, but rather is drawn out from our bones.

Although salt is important for us because it helps to maintain the pH balance of our blood, excessive salt intake can do us harm. Too much salt is unhealthful for other reasons. It may raise blood pressure, leading to heart and kidney problems, so a good approach would be to follow the American Heart Association guidelines and stay well under 2,000 milligrams of salt per day.

110. SHOULD I TAKE CALCIUM WITH OTHER FOODS OR ALONE?

If you are talking about eating calcium-rich foods with other foods, beware of eating them with fiber or with iron (see the answers to Questions 104 and 105). If you are talking about calcium supplements, there is no general medical consensus. Some doctors advise taking them with food; others say to take calcium separately. I still prefer to take mine at night when there is a minimum of interference with absorption from other foods or elimination of calcium through more frequent urinating, as might be the case during the day as a result of fluid consumption. However, avoid taking more than 500 to 600 milligrams at one time. We absorb calcium best if it is taken in small amounts throughout the day. Another tip: If you try to take it at the same times each day, you're less likely to forget to do so.

111. CAN ANYTHING BE DONE TO HELP ME WITH THE NAUSEA, GAS, AND BLOATING I GET WHEN I TAKE CALCIUM SUPPLEMENTS?

Some calcium supplements stimulate gastric acid secretions, wreaking havoc in our digestive tract. This is probably a preparation or dosage problem. Sometimes switching to a different form of calcium can help; so can increasing the dosage more slowly or dividing it more evenly throughout the day. Sometimes switching to a calcium-based antacid tablet will help, soothing the digestive tract and providing calcium at the same time.

112. IS IT TRUE THAT I SHOULD TAKE VITAMIN D TO HELP MY BODY ABSORB CALCIUM?

It is true that your body cannot absorb or use calcium without vitamin D. The RDA for vitamin D is 400 International Units (I.U.). Luckily, in most places in the United States we get enough vitamin D from the sunshine we are exposed to just going about our normal routine— thirty to sixty minutes of sunshine daily. In addition, most multivitamins include 400 milligrams of vitamin D. So does a quart of milk. So unless a person is house-bound or lives in a part of the world that lacks sunshine for prolonged periods, no additional vitamin D is necessary. Vitamin D helps to maintain the calcium and phosphorus levels in our bloodstream, which is beneficial, but too much vitamin D can draw calcium from our bones.

113. LATELY I HAVE SEEN THE VALUE OF VITAMIN D_3 MENTIONED IN ARTICLES ABOUT PRESERVING BONE. SHOULD I BE TAKING IT?

You may be referring to a study from Lyon, France, that was reported in the *New England Journal of Medicine*, December 3, 1992. The study, by Marie C. Chapuy, Ph.D., Monique E. Arlot, M.D., Francis DuBoeuf, Ph.D., and others, reported that after eighteen months of daily supplements of 1.29 milligrams of elemental calcium and 800 International Units (I.U.) of vitamin D_3 (cholecalciferol), there was a small decrease in hip fractures and other nonvertebral fractures in elderly women. The 3,270 women studied were between the ages of sixty-nine and one hundred six. The importance of these results is that they demonstrate that it may never be too late to prevent hip fractures. More research needs to be done before vitamin D_3 is available to us.

114. HOW MANY TUMS WOULD I HAVE TO TAKE IN A DAY TO MEET MY CALCIUM REQUIREMENTS?

That depends on your individual requirements based on your age and stage of life and from what other sources you get your calcium. For example, suppose you were trying to achieve a 1,000-milligram per day intake of calcium. Remember our earlier equation: If you drink an eight-ounce glass of skim milk you would ingest about 300 milligrams of calcium; add to that an eight-ounce container of nonfat yogurt at 350 milligrams of calcium. That's 650 milligrams already. Let's pretend that that is all the calcium you consume each day. If you then took two Tums, which contain roughly 200 milligrams of elemental calcium each, you would not only meet, but exceed your daily intake requirements by 50 milligrams. It's a numbers game, and you can be the winner!

115. I HAVE KIDNEY PROBLEMS AND A TENDENCY TO MAKE KIDNEY STONES TRIGGERED BY CALCIUM. WHAT ELSE CAN I DO TO FULFILL MY NEED FOR CALCIUM?

This is a situation that was covered briefly in Question 107 in this chapter. The answer remains: Discuss it with your doctor.

116. DO MEN HAVE THE SAME CALCIUM REQUIREMENTS AS WOMEN?

Although most medical research has been done with men, osteoporosis research is one area that has largely dealt with women. Very little is known of osteoporosis in men, although five million men each year fall victim to this disease. Remember that men have more bone mass to start out with than women do and that they lose it more slowly than we do. Men require calcium, too, and physicians assure me that the same diet, exercise, drug-intake, and substance-abuse admonitions apply to men as well. For women—and for men—it is a matter of taking action to prevent bone loss.

There is a Broadway musical that made its way to the United States from London a number of years ago that I particularly loved. It is called *The Roar of the Greasepaint— the Smell of the Crowd,* The lyrics of one song in particular fill my mind as I write this chapter—probably because it is about taking charge of your own destiny.

It isn't enough to stand here
Saying that life is grand here
Waiting for something good to turn up.

Leslie Bricusse and Anthony Newley,
"It Isn't Enough."©

Seven Ways in Seven Days to Pack Calcium into Your Diet

Here are seven days' worth of calcium-packed menu and snack ideas. All items are interchangeable among these suggested meals, and these calcium-rich foods can be combined with other food items and added to your daily eating plans.

When preparing these sample meals, reduced fat or nonfat or cholesterol-free products can often be substituted without sacrificing calcium content (and may be even higher in calcium). For example, 1 ounce of Alpine Lace Swiss cheese provides 200 milligrams of calcium, and ¾ ounce of Formagg (no cholesterol) provides 250 millligrams. A switch to Lite sour cream still offers 40 milligrams of calcium per ounce. However, 1 ounce of Borden's American cheese provides 150 milligrams of calcium, while 1 ounce of Borden's Lite or Fat-Free American cheese provides 200 milligrams.

Just a reminder—your target daily calcium consumption should be

- 1,500 milligrams if you are postmenopausal and are *not* taking estrogen;
- 1,000 milligrams if you are premenopausal or postmenopausal and *are* taking estrogen;
- 1,200 milligrams if you are pregnant or breastfeeding.

Throughout, unless otherwise specified, quantities should be considered to be an average serving. Please note that these calcium values are approximate inasmuch as recipes can vary and sizes of foods can vary as well.

SEVEN CALCIUM-RICH BREAKFASTS	
MENU SELECTION	MILLIGRAMS OF CALCIUM
Day One	
6 ounces of calcium-fortified orange juice	200
1 plain English muffin	92
2 tablespoons of jam	8
1–2 cups coffee or tea with ¼ cup milk	75
Day Two	
Quaker Instant Oatmeal or Total dry cereal (or check other brands)	200
½ cup skim milk	150
1 large orange	56
1–2 cups coffee or tea with ¼ cup milk	75
Day Three	
2 Aunt Jemima frozen waffles	100
2 tablespoons pure maple syrup	65
1 banana, sliced, honey, and ½ cup nonfat yogurt	200–225
1–2 cups coffee or tea with ¼ cup milk	75

What Kinds of Foods Can Protect Bones?

Day Four

Savory Cheese Toast: Top 2 slices of bread with a mixture of ½ cup ricotta cheese, beaten egg white, sugar, and cinnamon; broil.	400
1–2 cups coffee or tea with ¼ cup milk	75

Day Five

⅓ cup low-fat granola with 1 apple, diced, and ⅔ cup plain low-fat yogurt	275–300
1–2 cups coffee or tea with ¼ cup milk	75

Day Six

Breakfast Shake: Combine in a blender 1 cup of milk with 1 banana, ½ cup strawberries, and a teaspoon or so of wheat germ (optional).	325

Day Seven

3 4-inch pancakes from a mix (Aunt Jemima Buttermilk or Mrs. Butterworth's Old-Fashioned)	150–250
2 tablespoons of pure maple syrup	65
1 cup of strawberries	21
1–2 cups coffee or tea with ¼ cup milk	75

* In any of the breakfasts, you may substitute low-cal hot chocolate for the coffee or tea (Swiss Miss or Carnation) which provides 80–150 mg of calcium.

CALCIUM-RICH BREAKFAST-ON-THE-RUN	
MENU SELECTION	**MILLIGRAMS OF CALCIUM**
Carnation Instant Breakfast	400
Plain Nonfat Yogurt (with a half cup of raspberries)	414
Instant Oatmeal Packet (with hot water)	150–200

SEVEN CALCIUM-RICH LUNCHES	
MENU SELECTION	**MILLIGRAMS OF CALCIUM**
Day One	
2 tortillas topped with bean dip, ½ cup of chopped cooked broccoli, diced tomato, and 1 ounce of low-fat mozzarella cheese, broiled	300
1 large orange	56
Day Two	
Salmon salad in pita pocket (3 ounces pink salmon mashed with the bones and 2 tablespoons of plain yogurt)	330
½ large cantaloupe	45
1 8-ounce glass skim milk	300
Day Three	
1 cup of New England clam chowder (canned condensed milk added)	187

1 cup steamed green beans (as salad ingredient)	62
Chocolate pudding (1 cup, from mix, using skim milk)	300

Day Four

1 large baked sweet potato	50
topped with ½ cup of steamed broccoli and	68
1 ounce melted Swiss cheese	272
1 6-ounce glass calcium-fortified orange juice	200

Day Five

Savory Cheese Toast (see Day Four breakfast, flavored with fines herbs)	400
1 wedge watermelon	30

Day Six

3–4 ounces of canned sardines, with bones	300–450
6 black olives	20
French bread, 2 slices	30
1 cup diced papaya	50

Day Seven

1 cup low-fat cottage cheese	150
Carrot sticks (2 carrots)	55
1 loaf pita toast	60
½ large cantaloupe	45

SEVEN CALCIUM-RICH DINNERS	

MENU SELECTION	MILLIGRAMS OF CALCIUM
Day One	
2 cups cooked pasta with 1 cup cooked broccoli	450
4 tablespoons Parmesan cheese	300
Romaine lettuce salad with yogurt-based dressing (2 tablespoons plain yogurt)	40
½ cup ice milk	85–140
Day Two	
Stir-fried chicken (3–4 ounces) made with 1 cup bok choy	265
and ½ cup tofu, diced firm	258
1 cup steamed rice, any variety	21
½ cup cooked rhubarb (with lemon)*	174

Day Three

4 ounces broiled fish	40–60
1 cup cooked spinach (with lemon)*	244
Baked potato with plain yogurt topping (¼ cup)	100–110
1 cup rice pudding	260

Day Four

4 ounces shrimp on brochette	55
(eat the shrimp tails to pack in more calcium!)	250
Pear watercress salad (½ pear and 2 ounces watercress)	50
2 slices French bread	30
1 wedge pumpkin pie	58

Day Five

1 cup macaroni and cheese (2 ounces Cheddar)	400
1 cup collard greens, frozen cooked (with lemon)	360
1 cup blackberries	46

Day Six

Cheese pizza (⅓ of a 12-inch pie)	260
Green salad with yogurt dressing (2 tablespoons plain yogurt)	20
½ cup serving of frozen yogurt, flavored	80–150

Day Seven

4 ounces roast pork loin	10
1 baked large sweet potato	60
1½ cups steamed broccoli	270
Chocolate pudding (1 cup, from mix, using skim milk)	300

* When serving rhubarb and spinach (or other vegetables containing oxalates—see Question 73), serve with lemon because the lemon counteracts the effects of oxalic acid.

A BAKER'S DOZEN OF CALCIUM-RICH SNACKS

MENU SELECTION	MILLIGRAMS OF CALCIUM
1 cup nonfat flavored yogurt	350
1 medium orange	56
3 figs, dried	81
Raw vegetables with ¼ cup herbed nonfat yogurt and part-skim ricotta	200
Yogurt shake (8 ounces plain yogurt plus your favorite fruits)	350–450
1 ounce almonds	70
6 Hershey's Kisses (1 ounce milk chocolate)	53
½ large cantaloupe	45
4 caramels	55
1 frozen pudding bar or pop	80

1 cup buttermilk	300
1 4-ounce container pudding, packaged, Jell-O or Hershey's	80–100
1 8-ounce glass skim milk	300

HELPFUL HINTS

Serve rhubarb and spinach (and other vegetables containing oxalates) with lemon, which counteracts the effects of the oxalic acid (see Question 73).

When making soup, use the bones and add ¼ cup vinegar. The vinegar will dissolve calcium out of the bone and into the soup, adding calcium with no change in flavor. One pint of soup will then have the calcium content of 1 quart of milk.

Use tofu in place of chicken, meat, or fish in stir-fries, soups, and salads. Four ounces of tofu (the kind processed with a calcium salt) equals 250–300 milligrams of calcium.

Instead of butter, shake some Parmesan cheese on vegetables and popcorn. Four tablespoons equals 276 milligrams of calcium.

Add nonfat condensed or powdered milk to cream soups, sauces, and gravies. One teaspoon equals 50 mg of calcium.

CHAPTER 8

~

Can Hormone Replacement Therapy Help?

How many times have you been driving, and thought for a moment that the car in front of you was on automatic pilot, because you couldn't see the head of the person who appeared to be at the wheel? Then, as you moved beside the car, you realized that the woman (or man) was looking out of the windshield *through* the steering wheel, rather than over it. A loss of height, due to osteoporosis, is probably the culprit, as vertebral fractures shorten the spine.

A loss of height and a deformity in posture are just the external manifestations of osteoporosis. Internal organs may be cramped as the rib cage crowds down upon the hip bones, even making breathing difficult in extreme cases. And, all the while, the bones are becoming more porous and thin as demineralization occurs.

117. CAN HORMONE REPLACEMENT THERAPY HELP TO PROTECT MY BONES?

Yes, it can, according to Charles H. Chesnut III, M.D., director of the Osteoporosis Research Center, University of Washington Medical Center, Seattle. Dr. Chesnut believes that ERT is "the only proven preventive for postmenopausal osteoporosis." Dr. Chesnut is also a professor in the fields of medicine, radiology, nutritional services, and orthopedics, and he is a consultant to the National Institutes on Aging, and serves on the board of trustees of the National Osteoporosis Foundation. I feel very fortunate to serve frequently with Dr. Chesnut on panels about menopause and osteoporosis, because I know that with his expertise and cutting-edge knowledge, we are providing the women and men in our audiences with the best and the latest information about postmenopausal osteoporosis.

"The good news in 1992 is that this is a preventable, and, to a certain extent, a treatable disorder," said Dr. Chesnut as he began his talks last year. "We have a common and expensive problem," he continues. Then he discusses the statistics that I related earlier in this book—the twenty-five million cases of osteoporosis in 1990, the 1.5 million fractures both of the spine, or vertebrae, and the hip, and a cost that is now in excess of ten billion dollars per year.

Postmenopausal women are at the greatest risk for

153

osteoporosis, since with menopause, the ovaries stop making estrogen, which has a direct metabolic influence on the bones. Estrogen virtually slows down the rate of bone loss. With that braking action gone, bone loss occurs more quickly for the first seven to ten years after menopause, usually resuming its normal rate of loss after that period. By then, a postmenopausal woman who is at risk but is not on estrogen replacement therapy (ERT) may have lost approximately 30 percent of her skeleton.

118. When should I start ert or hrt?

According to Dr. Chesnut, "If estrogen replacement therapy is instituted soon after the onset of menopause, much of the bone loss, and subsequent fractures, may be prevented." He added: "Approximately one of every two women in the United States over the age of fifty may be at risk." Dr. Chesnut also believes that ERT or HRT may be valuable for women even when it is started later in life.

The first study to examine the effects of hormone therapy on older women was conducted at the University Hospital in Uppsala, Sweden, by Dr. Tord Naessen and colleagues and was reported in the *Annals of Internal Medicine*. It found that hormone replacement therapy produced a 60 percent reduction in the risk of hip fracture, no matter whether women used ERT (estrogen alone, usually because their uterus has been surgically removed) or HRT (estrogen combined with progestin because their uterus is intact). This study, reviewed in a *New York Times* article, July 16, 1990, suggests that hormone therapy may be far more powerful in maintaining the strength of the bones when it is started immediately at menopause, rather than over the age of sixty. Yet it still showed a 60 percent reduction in risk in older women. In commenting on the study, other experts in the field agreed that although maximum benefit may be derived from the timely start of hormone replacement therapy, women at any age who are at risk for osteoporosis probably will still benefit.

Bone loss can be dealt with in myriad ways when we're younger and aware of our risk factors and are willing to change our life-styles for the better. Once we enter the premenopausal or menopausal age range (ages forty-five to fifty-five, on average), women no longer have the luxury of having time on their side. When we're premenopausal or menopausal our options become more limited. In such cases, Dr. Chesnut indicates, estrogen replacement therapy may be our most important ally.

119. DOES ESTROGEN REPLACEMENT THERAPY SLOW OR STOP BONE LOSS?

Estraderm (the patch), Premarin, Estrace, and Ogen (oral preparations), are approved by the FDA for the prevention of osteoporosis. Applications are pending for these and others drugs to be approved for the treatment of osteoporosis, as well. That has not occurred as of this writing; however, it seems logical as studies point soundly in that direction.

Remember that osteoporosis occurs as the result of an abnormality in the bone remodeling process. In the seven to ten years immediately following menopause, our bone formation process does not keep pace with our bone loss. The perfect treatment, if discovered, would stop or slow bone loss and speed bone formation. "In 1992, we still don't have a single medication that can do both," reports Dr. Chesnut, "but we do have a number that can do one or the other."

120. Is lack of estrogen absolutely proven to be connected to osteoporosis?

Yes, it is, and that is why when estrogen production stops at menopause, women's bone loss accelerates, often rising from the 1 percent per year that is typical in aging to 3 percent per year or even more. Much is unknown about the physiological mechanisms by which this actually occurs. Some fairly recent data from a Mayo Clinic study using the estrogen patch (and reported in the *Annals of Internal Medicine*) demonstrated clearly that in women who already have osteoporosis—and even in some who have suffered fractures—an improvement in bone mass at the spine, and a lesser amount in the wrist and the hip, may follow the use of the estrogen patch. Other studies show that oral preparations of estrogen work the same way. This is heartening information!

121. ALONG WITH HRT OR ERT, WHAT ELSE SHOULD I DO TO PROTECT MY BONES?

Calcium is very important and, as we discussed, every woman should consume between 1,000 and 1,500 milligrams per day. Weight-bearing exercise is important and should be incorporated into life-style, but it is estrogen that cannot only prevent osteoporosis, but may also treat osteoporosis once we have it. The only other treatment that is approved to date by the FDA is salmon calcitonin, and it is approved in the United States only as an injectable. There are other drugs that are being developed, and we will discuss these in the next chapter. For now, let's focus on estrogen.

122. IS IT TRUE THAT UNLESS A POSTMENOPAUSAL WOMAN IS ON ERT, THE CALCIUM SUPPLEMENTS SHE TAKES WILL NOT BE ABSORBED AND USEFUL TO HER?

There are many studies that show that estrogen helps calcium work. Nothing in the area of osteoporosis research is static, however. Inasmuch as there is more research to be done in order to provide us with answers, and because the answer for each of us also depends on our own set of risk factors, medical history, and life-style, we need to discuss this matter with our physicians, who can help us to determine the risk/benefit ratio of ingesting calcium alone versus taking calcium and estrogen.

123. IF A POSTMENOPAUSAL WOMAN HAS A HIGH BONE-MINERAL DENSITY, IS ESTROGEN REPLACEMENT THERAPY STILL APPROPRIATE, SINCE ONLY ONE OUT OF TWO WOMEN EXHIBIT SYMPTOMS OF OSTEOPOROSIS?

Osteoporosis is called a silent disease because there literally are no symptoms. Either you learn that you have the disease from a bone-density test or you learn the sad truth after you suffer your first fracture. Here again, you must work in concert with your doctor. If your present high bone density has been determined by a bone-density test; if you have none of the other risk factors that can alter the strength of your bones; if you are ingesting enough calcium (1,500 milligrams per day is recommended after menopause), and if your exercise program includes the appropriate amount of weight-bearing exercise—then perhaps not. Currently, it is believed that about one-third of women may not require estrogen for any reason. Maybe you are one of them. But what if the cardioprotective effects of estrogen are proven without a doubt? Then ERT may be appropriate for you as well. Those are all factors that I encourage you to discuss with your physician.

124. SHOULD A WOMAN IN HER EIGHTIES, WHO HAS NEVER BEFORE TAKEN ESTROGEN, START NOW FOR OS-TEOPOROSIS CONTROL?

It depends. If you have suffered no bone loss of any significance up to this point, as measured by a bone-density test, there is probably no point in changing whatever it is that you do. I am assuming that you are a woman who has no risk factors that have affected you in any way and that your life-style works well for your skeletal health. By that, I mean that I hope you are consuming about 1,500 milligrams of calcium per day (through your diet or through calcium supplementation) and walking wherever and whenever you can to gain weight-bearing exercise. However, if you have suffered significant bone loss, then perhaps your physician might want to consider ERT to prevent further loss. I suggest that you take this question up with your physician. From your question, though, it sounds to me as if you're one of the lucky women!

125. MY SISTER DIED OF BREAST CANCER AT AGE FORTY-EIGHT. MY MOTHER HAS OSTEOPOROSIS. SHE'S EIGHTY-NINE. I KNOW THAT ESTROGEN CAN PREVENT BONE

LOSS BUT I HEARD THAT IT CAN ENHANCE CANCER
GROWTH. I FEAR BREAST CANCER, BUT I ALSO DON'T
WANT TO END UP WITH A "DOWAGER'S HUMP" ON MY
BACK. IS IT SAFE FOR ME TO TAKE ESTROGEN?

We often hear physicians describe to us the risk/
benefit ratio of a course of medical action. This is a perfect
example of the need to weigh that ratio carefully. I know
that your physician will wish to discuss this dilemma with
you. So many factors must be taken into consideration.
Your doctor will want to study your risk factors for breast
cancer and for osteoporosis. A family history of breast
disease is a serious factor for 20 percent of all women who
develop breast cancer. Some studies indicate that ERT may
increase breast-cancer risk, but the degree to which it does
is not known. Heredity is known to play a leading role in
an even larger percentage of women who have osteoporosis. ERT is known to be preventive of osteoporosis.
Another consideration, particularly for osteoporosis, would
be the difference in your life-style in contrast to that of
your mother. For example, do you have a history of
consuming an appropriate amount of calcium each day?
Does your exercise program support your need for healthy,
strong bones? And do your life-style and medical history
include any activities that may diminish bone mass, such as
smoking, excessive ingestion of alcohol, protein, caffeine,

or colas, or do you need to take cortisone-like or excessive amounts of thyroid medications or any other drugs that can leach calcium from your bones or prevent calcium absorption? Only after a complete study of these and other medical factors can a decision be made by you and your doctor. If you do decide to go on ERT, remember that hormones are powerful drugs, and you should see your physician yearly for a check-up and mammogram and, perhaps, twice each year for a breast examination. In addition, you should practice breast self-examination each month and always quickly report any changes to your physician. There is so much research under way into breast cancer, osteoporosis, and other women's health issues that the best thing you can do is stay informed of current findings and discuss with your doctor how these findings might pertain to you.

126. DOES THE ESTROGEN PATCH PROVIDE THE SAME PROTECTION AGAINST OSTEOPOROSIS AS THE ESTROGEN PILLS?

A study conducted by B. Lawrence Riggs, M.D., at the Mayo Clinic, Rochester, Minnesota, and reported in 1991, demonstrated the long-term benefits of the estrogen patch as a preventive for postmenopausal bone loss which can lead to fractures. Oral medications, Premarin, Estrace, and Ogen, also have been approved by the FDA for that purpose.

127. EVEN THOUGH MY HOT FLASHES AND OTHER SYMPTOMS HAVE STOPPED, HOW DO I KNOW THAT MY BONES ARE PROTECTED BY THE AMOUNT OF ESTROGEN I TAKE?

That's an excellent question. My experience has been that if my screening bone-density test showed no bone loss, and if after taking ERT my symptoms disappeared, then I felt fairly reassured that my bones were stable. Of course, along with ERT I take the recommended amount of calcium for my age, at least 1,000 milligrams per day, and I exercise a minimum of four times a week, making sure to include weight-bearing exercise. In addition, my life-style does not include any foods, drinks, or medications that might hamper that stability. Nonetheless, after five years on ERT, I did request a follow-up bone-density test to assure me that I had not lost bone (I had actually gained a small amount).

128. ARE THERE ANY SIGNS THAT I SHOULD WATCH FOR THAT WOULD INDICATE THAT I'M EXPERIENCING BONE LOSS?

Although bone loss is silent, offering no apparent symptoms, there are some signs that may serve as clues to whether you should be concerned. Are you shrinking in height? Does your upper back seem to be rounding? Has a rather minor bump or fall caused you to fracture a bone? Do you have frequent episodes of acute back pain in the areas just above and below your waistline (medically called the upper lumbar and lower thoracic regions), during routine activities or at rest? I suggest that you check out any and all of these signs with your physician.

129. I HAD A HYSTERECTOMY AND HAD BOTH OVARIES REMOVED WHEN I WAS IN MY THIRTIES. I WAS THROWN INTO MENOPAUSE, BUT MY SYMPTOMS WEREN'T TOO BAD, SO I DIDN'T BEGIN ESTROGEN REPLACEMENT THERAPY. NOW I'M WORRIED ABOUT MY BONES. WHAT SHOULD I DO?

I suggest that you ask your physician for a bone-density test to see whether you've lost any bone in the interim and that you consider ERT, if you have suffered bone loss. Even if your bones are still strong, you might want to discuss ERT with your doctor, inasmuch as your surgical menopause deprived your body of your natural estrogen so early in your life.

Actually, there is good news about life-style changes that can prevent osteoporosis, if we heed it. It seems to me that it's a matter of the E's—educate ourselves, empower ourselves to seek and get good medical care, eat right, exercise, and, if we need it, take estrogen. Also, we need to have a physician who is our partner in our quest for good health:

> *We need a physician who is a skilled professional, paid at an appropriate level, and regarded with an appropriate degree of respect, nothing more and nothing less.*

> John M. Smith, M.D.,
> *Women and Doctors*
> (Atlantic Monthly Press, 1992).

CHAPTER 9

What Is the Best Treatment for Osteoporosis?

The best treatment for osteoporosis would be a therapy that can replace lost bone. At this time, the only preparation that is approved in the United States by the FDA for the treatment of osteoporosis is salmon calcitonin. We've discussed estrogen in Chapter Eight. Salmon calcitonin, which slows the breakdown of bone, is our other option, and in the United States it is approved only as an injectable at this time. Dr. Charles Chesnut explains that "Salmon calcitonin is a prepration, rather like insulin, so it has to be given by needle and syringe." In Europe, a salmon calcitonin nasal spray is being used as well. This form of treatment may become available in the United States at some time in the future. We'll talk more about salmon calcitonin later in this chapter.

So much more research needs to be done, but this is all we have at the moment. A background paper called *The Menopause, Hormone Therapy, and Women's Health*, issued by the Office of Technology Assessment of the 102nd Congress of the United States (1992), reports on the need for research in postmenopausal osteoporosis along with the need for research in menopause. It outlines the areas of research needed to answer such vital questions as: Is ERT as effective on the bones of the femur as it is on the vertebrae? What is the effect of longterm progestin on bone mass? What is the cumulative effect of starting and stopping ERT (which is what many women do because they are nervous about "interfering with nature")? Is there a cumulative effect of ERT in the prevention of bone loss, or does bone loss begin again when ERT is discontinued? Does a woman's age (or the number of years she is postmenopausal) determine how great her decreased bone mass will be? And is ERT effective in preventing additional bone loss and fractures in women over the age of sixty-five?

What *is* known is that estrogen helps calcium work for us in our bodies. Our need for calcium throughout life has been covered in Chapter Seven. As you know, we need 1,000 to 1,500 milligrams daily from adolescence through senescence. We continue to need that calcium in conjunction with any osteoporosis treatment modalities we may undergo. We need it whether we obtain calcium through our diet, through supplementation, or in a combination thereof. Our need for calcium simply doesn't ever diminish.

Our need to build bone through weight-bearing exercise, covered in Chapter Six, also is complementary to any osteoporosis treatment plan. The right exercise plan for you and the appropriate intensity of that plan really should be worked out with your physician (and she or he should be a doctor who specializes in the treatment of osteoporosis), and should depend upon the degree of bone loss you have sustained. Avoid inactivity, if at all possible.

Since, thankfully, the medical profession, through the media, has made us more aware of the longterm, late-life, debilitating effects of osteoporosis, an ever-increasing number of women are concerned with protecting themselves from this disease.

130. HOW CAN I BE SURE I'M GETTING ENOUGH VITAMIN D TO COMPLEMENT THE CALCIUM I CONSUME? HOW MUCH DO I NEED?

We need about 400 milligrams of Vitamin D each day, which we can acquire in a good multivitamin. Vitamin D is crucial to enable the calcium you consume to be absorbed in your intestines and, therefore, to be useful to you. In sunny climates, you probably get sufficient vitamin D through your skin. No, don't go out and sit in the sun and bake—that's not good for your skin, and the incidence of skin cancer is on the rise. Just thirty minutes of sun each day as you go about your normal daily activities will give you enough vitamin D. You may wish to review other information concerning vitamin D that appears in Chapter Seven.

131. WHAT EXACTLY IS SALMON CALCITONIN?

Calcitonin is one of our body's natural bone hormones, produced by special cells in the thyroid gland. It works with vitamin D and parathyroid hormone as a regulating agency in your body, setting up a series of controls for maintaining your calcium levels and your bone mass. Calcitonin is believed to be the natural hormone that keeps the osteoclasts (the bone-destroying "Pac-men," described in Chapter One) from breaking down too much bone. Accordingly, researchers sought a way to treat women with osteoporosis by using synthetic calcitonin. The kind of calcitonin presently approved for use in therapy is made from salmon, and in the United States, is administered by injection. The two brands currently on the market are Miacalcin and Calcimar.

132. I'VE READ OF THE RELATIVE EASE OF USING THE NASAL SPRAY OF CALCITONIN, AS IS AVAILABLE IN EUROPE, VERSUS HAVING INJECTIONS. WHAT'S HOLDING UP THE NASAL SPRAY BEING AVAILABLE HERE?

Salmon calciton administered by nasal spray has not yet been approved by the FDA for use in the United States, although studies have been conducted with it.

133. ONCE YOU HAVE OSTEOPOROSIS, CAN ANYTHING BE DONE TO REVERSE BONE LOSS?

As mentioned earlier, there are currently two approved treatments for halting bone loss—estrogen and salmon calcitonin, plus a number of experimental drugs. There are also some very recent and encouraging studies from New York University that demonstrate that weight-bearing exercise and calcium alone may build bone mass, even in older adults.

134. CAN THE RISK OF OSTEOPOROSIS BE CURTAILED ENOUGH WITH DIET AND EXERCISE TO ELIMINATE THE NEED FOR ESTROGEN?

That answer depends on the strength of your bones. If you have none, or very few, of the risk factors for osteoporosis, and if you are eating and drinking enough calcium-rich foods and are performing enough weight-bearing exercise, you probably are protected. To be certain, I would suggest a baseline bone-density test, so that you know for sure that you have suffered no bone loss. If no loss has occurred, then just keep up the good work!

135. CAN FLUORIDES HELP IN THE TREATMENT OF OSTEOPOROSIS?

Scientists continue to study fluorides in combination with calcium as a treatment for osteoporosis. It is known that fluoride therapy increases bone-mineral density by creating trabecular bone. Fluoride therapy usually includes vitamin D and calcium. However, the quality of the bone made with this type of therapy remains in question. Also, there are questions about dosage. Low doses of fluorides are shown to reduce fractures, but higher doses may actually increase fracture rates. The fluorides used for treating osteoporosis are not used in the same way as those sold over the counter as nutrients or those in our water, which help strengthen our teeth and prevent decay. Fluorides may cause side effects, including joint pain, stomach ulceration, nausea, and vomiting. Taking fluorides with meals can help avert side effects, and a new slow-release capsule which may help as well is under clinical trial. Experimental studies with fluoride supplements for bone strengthening are under way, some of which are being conducted at the National Institutes of Health. Use of fluorides as treatment for osteoporosis has not been approved by the FDA.

136. WHAT IS ETIDRONATE AND HOW IS IT USED TO TREAT OSTEOPOROSIS?

Etidronate is one of the bisphosphonates (also known as diphosphonates) that are currently in clinical trials. They are still experimental and not yet approved by the

What Is the Best Treatment for Osteoporosis?

FDA. According to a September 1992 program syllabus, *Clinical Management of the Patient with Osteoporosis,* edited by Murray J. Favus, M.D., professor of medicine and director of clinical research, University of Chicago School of Medicine, and member of the Scientific Advisory Board of the National Osteoporosis Foundation, "Pyrophosphate is a naturally occurring inhibitor of bone mineralization." Whether natural or synthetic, these pyrophosphatelike compounds work to prevent bone loss. There are a number of bisphosphonates under clinical investigation. Etidronate, however, was approved by the FDA in the 1970s as a treatment for Paget's disease, a condition in which there is an excessive amount of bone turnover, resulting in new bone that, although dense, is fragile.

137. IF ETIDRONATE WORKS, HOW SOON WILL BONE DENSITY BE RESTORED?

Studies have shown that after two years, etidronate can increase bone mineral density and decrease fracture rates. Several other bisphosphonates are under trial. According to Dr. Favus, "The initial studies of bisphosphonates in the prevention of osteoporotic fractures appear promising, but additional follow-up is necessary to determine whether the increased bone mass and decreased fracture rates are sustained."

138. IS THERE ANYTHING ELSE THAT'S IN THE RESEARCH PHASE THAT OFFERS HOPE FOR OSTEOPOROSIS TREATMENT AND BONE REPLACEMENT?

Medical research never stands still. A good rule of thumb, I think, is that if in the last two years you have not been reevaluated by your physician for whatever condition you might have, it's a good idea to go back to your doctor to find out what's new. In terms of the treatment for osteoporosis, any number of agents and protocols are being investigated. In addition to those discussed here—fluroides and bisphosphonates—studies are under way with vitamin D (calcitriol), thiazide diuretics, progestogens, anabolic steroids, and parathyroid hormone. There may be other agents being studied as well. Medicine continues to move forward!

139. IF I HAVE QUESTIONS ABOUT ADVANCES IN OSTEOPOROSIS TREATMENT, HOW CAN I FIND OUT WHAT'S NEW?

According to the NOF brochure, "The National Osteoporosis Foundation is the nation's leading resource for patients, health-care professionals, and organizations seeking up-to-date, medically sound information and program materials on the causes, prevention, and treatment of osteoporosis."

What Is the Best Treatment for Osteoporosis?

You can write to the NOF (see Appendix D) for information and publications.

A good long view is imperative when you are dealing with any illness. Hope is the ally of recovery, and it is knowledge and perseverance that can often help to determine our fate.

There is always so much trial and error in scientific research. One study shows us a direction; another refutes it. And so it goes. But we must never give up!

A thousand things advance; nine hundred and ninety-nine retreat; that is progress.

> Henri Frédéric Amiel,
> Swiss philosopher/poet,
> *Journal*, 1882–84.

Chapter 10

How Can I Keep Standing
Tall?

I met a woman in San Diego who shared an interesting story with me. I'll call her Kate. "Do you want to know how osteoporosis saved my life?" Kate offered. I smiled at this tall, attractive, well-dressed woman who stood before me. "Sure," I said. I was delighted with the prospect that she would share something positive or constructive about this destructive disease. She began:

I'm fifty-five years old, and I have osteoporosis. Before my bone-density test, just five years ago, I had a totally different life-style. It was then that I took myself to see a gynecologist because my menstrual cycle was goofy and I would break out into a sweat or chills for no reason at all.

The doctor examined me and explained that I might be going through menopause. He made some tests and asked me to call him in a few days. He also had me fill out and leave with his nurse a form that he had labeled a "life-style questionnaire." If this had been a graded test, let me tell you, I would have flunked. On it I had to admit that I still smoked cigarettes, enjoyed too many alcoholic beverages, and made up for their empty calories by filling up on diet soda each day. I rarely exercised and never thought about calcium. In addition, years ago some doctor gave me a thyroid medication that I had continued to take to that day.

The nurse called me a few days later and told me that the doctor would like to schedule a bone-density test for me because he had some concerns. She called it a DEXA. I agreed to go get it done and to come in for a follow-up visit.

When I showed up for the follow-up visit, my doctor showed real concern. He told me my blood test confirmed that I was menopausal, that my life-style self-evaluation indicated that I had programmed myself for a short life, and that my bone-density results showed that I had lost about 20 percent of my bone mass. WOW!

I panicked! Did he mean a short life, or life as a short person? I asked. "You could be facing either one or both," he said earnestly. Then he laid out a plan for my redemption.

I promised to quit smoking, limit alcohol intake, and give up soda—diet or otherwise. I agreed to be weaned off my thyroid medication, so that he could see whether I really required it. (My blood test had shown that my thyroid was too *active!*) Meanwhile, I promised to follow his chart of calcium-rich foods, buy a calcium supplement, and take in at least 1,000 milligrams of calcium each day. I also agreed to perform weight-bearing exercise in the prescribed amount (although at heart, I'm a couch potato). And I went on estrogen replacement therapy.

It's been five years since I cleaned up my life-style. What a difference there is in me! I feel charged with energy, and my figure is better than ever. More important, along with my last check-up I had another DEXA, and my bone loss has not only stopped, but it seems that I've added a little new bone as well. But the big point I want to make is that my osteoporosis scare made me take control of many other life-style factors—and change them for the better. I didn't want to have a short life!

I include Kate's story because I found it uplifting and inspiring. It's like that old, perhaps trite, saying: "What do you do if life hands you lemons? You make lemonade!"

There are so many reasons why we all have to take control of our health and our lives. Since medical science has created a longer life span for us, isn't it our responsibility to do everything in our power to make it a good long life—filled with good health and good times? At the conclusion of the talks I give around the country, I always express how I really feel about aging. I believe that your age is simply a number. That's all! I have friends in their thirties and friends who are in their eighties, and I think we're all the same age until one of us gets sick.

Now, let's cover the remaining questions that women asked as part of their top one hundred and fifty questions about osteoporosis. I saved these for last, because they are essentially wellness questions—questions that show women do want to take action to manage their health and their health care.

140. HOW IMPORTANT IS IT TO KNOW MY BONE DENSITY?

I think it is very important, because I am always convinced that we're better off when we know exactly where we are and what we've got to do. Reread the risk factors for osteoporosis in Chapter Three. If you have none, and have always, since youth, consumed an optimum amount of calcium and performed weight-bearing exercise, and you take estrogen, you probably have nothing to be concerned about. Nonetheless, I think it's a good idea at midlife to make sure your bones are healthy and strong by having your bone density checked—at least once.

141. WHAT EXACTLY IS PEAK BONE MASS?

The term *peak bone mass* refers to the maximum amount of bone that you will ever have. Earlier in this book we discussed how you can usually continue to build bone until about the age of thirty or thirty-five. After that, you can work to maintain bone or perhaps, as some recent studies show, rebuild just a little.

142. HOW DO I BUILD PEAK BONE MASS WHEN I'M IN MY TEENS, TWENTIES, AND THIRTIES TO PREVENT LOSING MUCH BONE AS I AGE?

Now that you know more about your bones and have learned how the bone remodeling process works, you can work to build greater bone mass by adding calcium-rich foods to your diet, by adding weight-bearing activities to your exercise program, and by eliminating smoking and products or medications that leach calcium out of your bones. In your teens, twenties, and early thirties, these activities will enable you to work toward building a higher peak bone mass, so that when in the normal course of aging you begin to lose bone, you'll be losing it from a higher peak and, thus, have more bone left after the loss.

143. WHAT CAN WOMEN DO TO CONVINCE ALL THE YOUNG FEMALES IN THEIR FAMILIES ABOUT THE LIFE-STYLE CHANGES THAT THEY NEED TO ADOPT IN THEIR TEENS, TWENTIES, AND THIRTIES IN ORDER TO PREVENT OS-TEOPOROSIS LATER IN LIFE?

This is one of the most common questions raised at programs at which I speak. I think the answer to this question could stem the epidemic of osteoporosis-caused hip fracture that is predicted along with our longer life spans. The best way we can teach is by example and explanation. It is worth it to interfere in our young relatives' lives to encourage them to understand how the self-help role that they play now can positively influence their health, and may prolong their lives. If young women in their teens, twenties, and thirties heed the advice about increasing their calcium consumption to 1,000 milligrams per day, every day, and planning and executing an exercise program that affords them flexibility, aerobic, and weight-bearing exercises, and if they eliminate the deleterious habits that can thin their bones and shrink their life spans, they can look forward to long, healthy, active lives. Sometimes, simply by sharing something you've read in a book, magazine, or newspaper article, you can attune young women to the problem of osteoporosis and the solutions that can work for them.

144. I'M A TEENAGER AND I'M ALWAYS TRYING TO LOSE WEIGHT, SO I DRINK DIET SODAS TO FILL ME UP SO I WON'T EAT. HOW CAN I PROTECT MY BONES?

Forget the sodas and begin to drink water. Eight glasses of water per day tends to make you feel full, and also offers many other health benefits. Water can help your body metabolize stored fat. Feel bloated? Water is a natural diuretic and can flush your body to rid it of excess liquid. It also works to enhance muscle tone. Another benefit to your digestive system and complexion is that water helps your body get rid of toxins and waste.

Add eight ounces of nonfat yogurt and an eight-ounce glass of skim milk to your diet each day and you won't put on weight, but you will protect your bones. Both make excellent and filling snacks.

145. I'M IN MY LATE TWENTIES AND I EAT A CALCIUM-RICH DIET, BUT I'M HOLDING DOWN A PART-TIME JOB AT THE OFFICE AND A FULL-TIME JOB AT HOME MOTHERING ONE-YEAR-OLD TWIN DAUGHTERS. I JUST DON'T HAVE TIME TO GO TO THE GYM ANYMORE. HOW DO I PROTECT MY BONES?

I know you're busy, but not too busy to take those twins out walking in their stroller. Do that and walk briskly for twenty to thirty minutes at least three times a week, and the twins will get their outings while you protect your bones.

146. I JUST CELEBRATED MY THIRTY-FIFTH BIRTHDAY AND NOW YOU TELL ME THAT I MISSED THE OPPORTUNITY TO BUILD PEAK BONE MASS. WHAT SHOULD I DO?

Now is the perfect time for you to begin to maintain your bone mass, long before you enter the years of rapid bone loss that follow menopause. So start today to consume 1,000 to 1,200 milligrams of calcium each day; begin a weight-bearing exercise program; and alter your life-style by eliminating those substances that can draw calcium out of your bones. To begin today, you may wish to review Chapters Five through Seven.

147. I'M FIFTY-ONE YEARS OLD AND MY PERIODS ARE JUST BEGINNING TO GET ERRATIC. I THINK I'VE HAD A FEW NIGHT SWEATS. IF MENOPAUSE IS ON ITS WAY, HOW CAN I MAKE SURE I WON'T GET OSTEOPOROSIS?

Reread the risk factors for osteoporosis listed in Chapter Three. Do any of them pertain to you? When you go to see your physician about those quirky periods and night sweats, discuss your risk factors for osteoporosis (or your lack of them) at that time. Then, you and your doctor can determine whether your bone density should be tested and whether or when you should begin ERT. In the meantime, make sure you are getting 1,000 to 1,200 milligrams of calcium each day, that you are performing weight-bearing exercises, and that you are eliminating, wherever possible, substances that can speed up your bone loss.

148. I'M IN MY LATE SEVENTIES. I ALREADY HAVE OS-TEOPOROSIS. WHAT CAN I DO TO PREVENT FRACTURES?

Living with your own personal safety in mind is a key to living independently once you have osteoporosis. You need to do everything you can to prevent falls and strains to your back—both of which can result in fractures. Here are twelve tips for personal safety:

1. Religiously follow the exercise program that *your doctor recommends*. Exercise can increase the support that your muscles give your bones, as well as improve your balance and flexibility.
2. Be careful of medications that can dull your sense of balance.
3. Wear shoes that give you good support.
4. Put railings wherever you need them, particularly in the bathroom at the tub or shower, and at stairways. Use handrails wherever they are provided.
5. Avoid walking or doing physical work in areas that are poorly lighted.
6. Do not lift heavy objects.
7. Don't strain to open things, like a stuck door or window. Don't hesitate to ask for assistance.
8. Bend your knees and keep your back straight when you need to pick something up from the floor or any lower surface.
9. Don't climb on chairs, stools, or ladders to reach things in high places—ask for help. Keep frequently used items in easy-to-reach places.
10. Check the floors to make sure you have no loose rugs or mats and no dangling electrical or telephone cords

that can trip you. If you have a pet, always check to see where it is, so that you don't trip over a pet snoozing in your path.

11. If you get up at night, turn on the lights. Don't walk around in the dark. Use night lights. If you're afraid you'll wake your mate, keep a bright flashlight next to the bed.

12. Remember to use caution in your everyday tasks—every day.

149. IS OSTEOPOROSIS A NORMAL PART OF GROWING OLD?

Absolutely not. The life-style changes that have been discussed throughout this book can help you to protect your bones, maintain your bone mass, and live better while you're living longer. An explicit goal we all share is to remain independent throughout our lives. We can maintain our independence by continuing to educate ourselves about how our bodies age and by promoting life-styles that can benefit us. Let's start now!

150. HOW DO I FIND THE RIGHT DOCTOR TO HELP ME MEET MY GOALS FOR MAINTAINING MY GOOD HEALTH AND STRONG BONES?

Do a little worthwhile research. Ask your friends, family members, neighbors, and coworkers for the name of a doctor they might know who is interested in the care of women—and who practices preventive medicine. Call your local hospital and ask the same question. List all the names that you get. Soon you'll have lists from your various sources. See which names keep appearing on the lists. Those good names, like cream, will rise to the top of the list.

Then make appointments with and interview the two or three doctors who are at the top of your list. When you call for your appointment, explain that you're coming for a consultation and ask for, and be prepared to pay for, some extra time. (The future quality of your health may depend on making that small investment. In the long run, it's well worth it.)

At your consultation appointment, ask the physician if she or he is interested in preventive health care of women as we age. Ask what percentage of the patients in the practice are about your age. The answers to those questions will help you learn whether this is the doctor for you. Describe your good-health goals and find out whether the doctor's approach to maintaining healthy bones—diet, weight-bearing exercise, calcium supplementation, estrogen replacement therapy (or HRT)—is in concert with yours.

Choose the physician with whom you feel you can forge a partnership and work to preserve or enhance your good health and in whom you feel the most confident. Your choice will probably reflect your physician's level of interest in helping you stay healthy!

All of us, regardless of age, want to prevent osteoporosis. I, for one, heed all the good-health advice that I can get. I hope that you, too, will work toward a good, long, and independent life by fulfilling the following Edicts:

Educate yourself about ways to preserve your good health
Empower yourself to get proper medical care
Eat right
Exercise and, if appropriate for you, take
Estrogen

A Final Note:
Write to Me, Talk to Me

In *150 Most-Asked Questions About Menopause*, I invited open lines of communication between me and my readers. Since its publication, I have heard from thousands of women—some sharing their experiences, others looking for help and advice. I also continue to speak to large groups of women and men at the programs in which I participate, as well as through the media. I hope that I have helped women both in understanding menopause and osteoporosis and in empowering them to get what they need from the health-care delivery system. I know their letters have helped me to keep abreast of what women really want to know.

With the publication of *150 Most-Asked Questions About Osteoporosis*, I again offer open lines of communication with my readers. From this relationship, I hope we can all learn more about how to prepare for and live a first-rate second half of adult life. Taking care of your medical needs requires a medical doctor, and I hope I have encouraged you to forge a partnership with the doctor who is right for you. But we may wish to share myriad other points of information and hints about life-style changes that have worked for us. We all want to keep informed about medical and nonmedical self-help methods.

My address is available to you, and I am delighted to receive your suggestions, comments, and questions. I have heard from so many women, and I know that I have a lot of new friends all around the country. I can't promise to respond to each of your letters individually, but I can promise that you will receive a card or note letting you know that the information you have shared is in the hopper of good ideas for my next consumer book.

Please do not include requests for referrals to physicians in your area. But do check Appendix D for other organizations, both national and, perhaps, in your area, that can provide resource information for you. Some may even be able to assist with physician referrals. These organizations usually prefer that you write to them rather than call.

To keep up to date on osteoporosis, you may wish to join the National Osteoporosis Foundation. Write them for membership information. The address can be found in Appendix D.

If you wish to stay in touch and share your thoughts and ideas with me in the hope of helping other women, please write to me at the following address:

A Final Note: Write to Me, Talk to Me

Ruth S. Jacobowitz
5 Longmeadow Lane
Cleveland, OH 44122

Thank you for joining my consumer research project that is focused on continuing to learn and to share "what women really want to know"!

Ruth S. Jacobowitz

Afterword

In 1993 a number of therapies are available for preventing and treating osteoporosis, including the FDA-approved therapies, estrogen, and synthetic salmon calcitonin. However, the decade of the 1990s promises continual development of additional therapies for this common and expensive disease, including the bisphosphonates (etidronate, alendronate, residronate, tiludronate, and possibly pamidronate), the newer congeners of vitamin D with greater specificity for bone formation and lesser specificity for gut calcium absorption, the nonsteroidal anti-inflammatory medications, and possibly stimulators of bone formation such as various cytokines (TGF-β, insulin-like growth factors, etc.). In addition, in the future there will be increased attention to calcium, particularly for younger individuals to attain greater peak bone mass, and increased attention to the advantages of exercise to promote good bone health.

The decade of the 1990s is a most exciting time for the

treatment of osteoporosis; information for the consumer, such as is imparted in this book, will have definite value in affecting this most common and expensive disease, osteoporosis.

> Charles H. Chesnut III, M.D.
> Professor, Medicine, Radiology
> Director, Osteoporosis Research Center
> University of Washington Medical Center
> Seattle, Washington

Appendix A

Recommended Reading and References

Appleton, Nancy, Ph.D. *Healthy Bones: What You Should Know About Osteoporosis.* Garden City Park, NY: Avery Publishing, 1991.

Beard, Mary, M.D., and Lindsay Curtis, Ph.D. *Menopause and the Years Ahead.* Tucson: Fisher Books, 1991.

Boston Women's Health Collective, The. *The New Our Bodies, Ourselves.* New York: Touchstone/Simon and Schuster, 1984.

Cobb, Janine O'Leary. *Understanding Menopause.* Toronto, Canada: Key Porter Books Limited, 1989.

Cooper, Kenneth H. *The New Aerobics for Women.* New York: Bantam Books, 1988.

————. *Preventing Osteoporosis: The Kenneth Cooper Method.* New York: Bantam Books, 1989.

Appendix A

Doress, Paula Brown, and Diana Laskin Siegal. *Ourselves, Growing Older*. New York: Simon and Schuster, 1987.

Fardon, David F., M.D. *Osteoporosis: Your Head Start on the Prevention and Treatment of Brittle Bones*. Los Angeles: The Body Press, 1987.

Goulder, Lois, and Leo Lutwak, M.D., Ph.D. *The Strong Bones Diet*. Gainesville, FL: Triad Publishing Company, 1988.

Hausman, Patricia, and Judith Benn Hurley. *The Healing Foods*. Emmaus, PA: Rodale Press, 1989.

Jacobowitz, Ruth S. *150 Most-Asked Questions About Menopause: What Women Really Want to Know*. New York: Hearst Books, 1993.

Lark, Susan M., M.D. *The Menopause Self-Help Book*. Berkeley, CA: Celestial Arts, 1990.

Madaras, Lynda, and Jane Patterson, M.D., with Peter Schick, M.D. *Womancare: A Gynecological Guide to Your Body*. New York: Avon Books, 1981.

Mayes, Kathleen. *Osteoporosis: Brittle Bones and the Calcium Crisis*. Santa Barbara, CA: Pennant Books, 1986.

Melpomene Institute for Women's Health Research, The. *The Bodywise Woman*. New York: Prentice Hall Press, 1990.

Appendix A

National Osteoporosis Foundation, The. *Boning Up on Osteoporosis*. 1991. (Copies are $2.00. For copies, write to: The National Osteoporosis Foundation, 1150 17th Street NW, Suite 500, Washington, DC 20036-4603.)

———. *Facts About Osteoporosis, Arthritis, and Osteoarthritis*. 1991.

———. *The Older Person's Guide to Osteoporosis*. 1991.

———. *Stand Up to Osteoporosis*. 1992.

Osteoporosis Society of Canada, The. P.O. Box 280, Station Q, Toronto, Ontario M4T 2MI.

Prevention Magazine. *Future Youth: How to Reverse the Aging Process*. Emmaus, PA: Rodale Press, 1987.

———. *Prevention's Book of Home Remedies: Over 200 Fast-Action Remedies*. Emmaus, PA: Rodale Press, 1990.

Rozek, Jan, R.N. *Keys to Understanding Osteoporosis*. Hauppauge, NY: Barron's Educational Series, 1992.

Shangold, Mona, M.D., and Gabe Mirkin, M.D. *The Complete Sports Medicine Book for Women*. New York: Fireside Books, 1985.

Shephard, Bruce D., M.D., and Carroll A. Shephard, R.N.,

Ph.D. *The Complete Guide to Women's Health*. New York: Plume/Penguin, sec. rev. ed., 1990.

Shock, Nathan W., Richard C. Greulich, Reubin Andres, et al. *Normal Human Aging: The Baltimore Longitudinal Study of Aging*. U.S. Dept. of Health and Human Services, 1984.

Smith, John M., M.D. *Women and Doctors*. New York: The Atlantic Monthly Press, 1992.

Tapley, Donald F., M.D., Thomas Q. Morris, M.D., Lewis P. Rowland, M.D., et al. *The Columbia University College of Physicians and Surgeons Complete Home Medical Guide*. New York: Crown, 1989.

Thompson, D.S., M.D., consulting editor. *EveryWoman's Health: The Complete Guide to Body and Mind by 15 Women Doctors*. Garden City, NY: 1990.

University of California, Berkeley. *The Wellness Encyclopedia*. Boston: Houghton Mifflin, 1991.

U.S. Department of Health and Human Services, Public Health Service, and National Institutes of Health. *Osteoporosis: Cause, Treatment, Prevention*. May, 1986. NIH Publication No. 86-2226.

———. *Osteoporosis*. April, 1989. NIH Publication No. 89-2893. (For copies, write to: Clinical Center Communications, National Institutes of Health, 9000 Rockville Pike, Building 10, Room 1C255, Bethesda, MD 20892.)

Utian, Wulf, M.D., Ph.D., and Ruth S. Jacobowitz. *Managing Your Menopause*. New York: Fireside/Simon and Schuster, 1990.

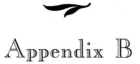

Appendix B

Other Professional Sources

American Health. "Estrogen Up in Smoke." December, 1992; Vol. XI, No. 10, p. 8.

———. "More Calcium for Kids." November, 1992; Vol. XI, No. 9, p. 94.

The American Journal of Medicine. "Consensus Development Conference: Prophylaxis and Treatment of Osteoporosis." Conference report. January, 1991; Vol. 90, pp. 107–110.

Avioli, Louis V., M.D. "Osteoporosis Syndromes: Patient Selection for Calcitonin Therapy." *Geriatrics.* April, 1992; Vol. 47, No. 4, pp. 58–67.

———. "Therapeutic Endpoints in Osteoporosis." Proceedings of Calcimar Dialectic, a closed symposium, November 18–19, 1988.

Appendix B

Chapuy, Marie, Ph.D.; Monique E. Arlot, M.D.; Francois DuBoeuf, Ph.D.; et al. "Vitamin D_3 and Calcium to Prevent Hip Fractures in Elderly Women." *The New England Journal of Medicine*, December 3, 1992; Vol. 327, No. 23, pp. 1637–1642.

Chesnut, Charles H. III, M.D. "Osteoporosis and Its Treatment." *The New England Journal of Medicine*, February 6, 1992; Vol. 326, No. 6, pp. 406–407.

Consumer Reports. "Are You Eating Right?" October, 1992; Vol. 57, No. 10, pp. 644–651.

———. "Osteoporosis." Special report. October, 1984.

Drinkwater, Barbara L., Ph.D. "The Role of Exercise." *Menopause Management*, September/October, 1992; Vol. 1, No. 2, pp. 20–25.

Drug Topics. "Osteoporosis, The Bone-Crushing Ailment: What you should know." May 20, 1991; pp. 22–30.

Ettinger, Bruce, M.D.; Harry K. Genant, M.D.; Peter Steiger, Ph.D.; and Phillip Madvig, M.D. "Low-dosage Micronized 17B-estradiol Prevents Bone Loss in Postmenopausal Women." *American Journal of Obstetrics and Gynecology*, February, 1992; Vol. 166, No. 2, pp. 479–488.

Fogelman, I., B.Sc., F.R.C.P.; and P. Ryan, M.A., M.R.C.P. "Osteoporosis: A Growing Epidemic." *British Journal of Clinical Practice*, Autumn, 1991; Vol. 45, No. 3, pp. 189–196.

Fugh-Berman, Adriane, M.D., and Samuel Epstein, M.D. "Should Healthy Women Take Tamoxifen?" *The New England Journal of Medicine*, November 26, 1992; Vol. 327, No. 22, p. 1596.

Gennari, Carlo; Donato Agnusdei; Mario Montagnani; et al. "An Effective Regimen of Intranasal Salmon Calcitonin in Early Postmenopausal Bone Loss." *Calcified Tissue International*, April, 1992; Vol. 50, No. 4, pp. 381–383.

Gillespy, Thurman III, M.D.; and Marjorie P. Gillespy, M.D. "Osteoporosis." *Radiologic Clinics of North America*, January, 1991; Vol. 29, No. 1, pp. 77–82.

Herman, Robin. "The Silent Crippler." *Mirabella*, November, 1992; pp. 116–118.

JAMA. "At Third Meeting, Menopause Experts Make the Most of Insufficient Data." Vol. 268, No. 18, pp. 2483–2485.

Johnston, C. Conrad, Jr., M.D.; Judy Z. Miller, Ph.D., Charles W. Slemenda, Dr.P.H.; et al. "Calcium Supplementation and Increases in Bone Mineral Density in Children." *The New England Journal of Medicine*, July 9, 1992; Vol. 327, No. 2, pp. 82–87.

Kaplan, Frederick S., M.D. "Osteoporosis/ Pathology and Prevention." *Clinical Symposia*, 1987; Vol. 39, No. 1.

Kaufman, Elizabeth. "Boning Up." *Self*, November, 1991; pp. 142–3, 178.

———. "The New Case for Woman Power." *The Good Health Magazine; New York Times*, April 28, 1991; pp. 18–22.

Lindsay, Robert, M.B., Ch.B., Ph.D. "Osteoporosis: Practical Aspects of Management." *Resident and Staff Physician*, June, 1991; Vol. 37, No. 6, pp. 17–23.

Lufkin, Edward G., M.D.; Heinz W. Wahner, M.D.; William M. O'Fallon, Ph.D.; et al. "Treatment of Postmenopausal Osteoporosis with Transdermal Estrogen." *Annals of Internal Medicine*, July 1, 1992; Vol. 117, No. 1, pp. 1–9.

Matkovic, Velimir, M.D., Ph.D. "Calcium Intake and Peak Bone Mass." *The New England Journal of Medicine*, July 9, 1992; Vol. 327, No. 2, pp. 119–120.

Mayo Clinic Health Letter. "Calcium and Osteoporosis." February, 1991; pp. 6–7.

———. "Estrogen Replacement Therapy." May, 1991; p. 7.

Miller, Paul D., M.D. "Early Diagnosis and Intervention are Goals in Osteoporosis Management." *Menopause Management*, July/August, 1992; Vol. 1, No. 1, pp. 25–32.

Nachtigall, Lila E., M.D.; and Margaret J. Nachtigall, M.D. "The Perimenopause and Vasomotor Symptoms." *Postgraduate Medicine*, August 22, 1990; special report, pp. 5–8.

National Osteoporosis Foundation. "Current Perspectives on Diagnosis, Prevention, and Treatment of Osteoporosis." Consensus statements, January, 1991.

———. "Physician's Resource Manual on Osteoporosis: A Decision-Making Guide." 1991.

Neer, Robert M., M.D.; Fournier, Albert, M.D.; and Jean Luc Sebert, M.D. "Calcitriol or Calcium for Postmenopausal Osteoporosis" (separate letters). *The New England Journal of Medicine*, July 23, 1992; Vol. 327, No. 4, p. 284.

Newsweek. "Menopause: The Search for Straight Talk and Safe Treatment," May 25, 1992, Vol. 119, No. 21, pp. 70–82.

Niewoehner, Catherine B., M.D. "Osteoporosis Management: Ten Questions Physicians Often Ask." *Consultant*, May, 1992; pp. 131–139.

Notelovitz, Morris, M.D., Ph.D. "Hormone Replacement Therapy in the Prevention of Cardiovascular Disease." *Postgraduate Medicine*, August 22, 1990; special report, pp. 23–32.

Nutrition Reviews. "Preventing Wintertime Bone Loss: Effects of Vitamin D Supplementation in Healthy Postmenopausal Women." February, 1992; Vol. 50, No. 2, pp. 52–54.

Office of Technology Assessment (United States Congress). Background paper: "The Menopause, Hormone Therapy, and Women's Health," May, 1992.

Papazian, Ruth. "Osteoporosis Treatment Advances." *FDA Consumer*, April, 1991; Vol. 25, No. 3, p. 32.

San Roman, Gabriel A., M.D.; and Howard L. Judd, M.D. "Adverse Effects of Hormone Replacement Therapy." *Postgraduate Medicine*, August 22, 1990; special report, pp. 39–46.

Schroeder, Patricia. "Women's Health: A Focus for the 1990s." *Women's Health Issues*, Spring 1992; Vol. 2, No. 1, pp. 1–2.

Smidt, Gary L., Ph.D., P.T.; Shen-Yu Lin, M.A., P.T.; Kathleen D. O'Dywer, M.A., P.T.; and Peter R. Blanpied, Ph.D., P.T. "The Effect of High-Intensity Trunk Exercise on Bone Mineral Density of Postmenopausal Women." *Spine*, March 17, 1992; Vol. 17, No. 3, pp. 280–285.

Smith, Roger. "Osteoporosis After 60." *British Medical Journal*, September 8, 1990; Vol. 301, No. 6750, pp. 452–453.

Steiniche, T.; C. Hasling; P. Charles; et al. "The Effects of Etidronate on Trabecular Bone Remodeling in Postmenopausal Spinal Osteoporosis: A Randomized Study Comparing Intermittent Treatment and an ADFR Regime." *Bone*, 1991; Vol. 12, pp. 155–163.

Studd, John; Timothy Garnett; and Michael Savvas. "Osteoporosis After 60." *British Medical Journal*, October 6, 1990; Vol. 301, No. 6755, p. 816.

Tilyard, Murray W., M.B., Ch.B; George F.S. Spears, M.Sc., B.A., B.Com.; Janet Thomson, R.G.O.N., R.M.; and Susan Dovey. "Treatment of Postmenopausal Osteoporosis with Calcitriol or Calcium." *The New England Journal of Medicine*, February 6, 1992; Vol. 326, No. 6, pp. 357–362.

Tosteson, Anna N.A., Sc.D.; Daniel I. Rosenthal, M.D.; L. Joseph Melton, III, M.D.; and Milton C. Weinstein, Ph.D. "Cost Effectiveness of Screening Perimenopausal White Women for Osteoporosis: Bone Densitometry and Hormone Replacement Therapy." *Annals of Internal Medicine*, October 15, 1990; Vol. 113, No. 8, pp. 594–603.

U.S. Department of Health and Human Services, Public Health Service, and National Institutes of Health. The Baltimore Longitudinal Study of Aging. "Older and Wiser." September, 1989. NIH Publication No. 89-2797.

————. (National Institute of Arthritis and Musculoskeletal and Skin Diseases). "Overview: HHS and Private Sector Efforts in Osteoporosis." 1991.

————. List of medical centers studying etidronate. September, 1990.

————. "Osteoporosis Research, Education and Health Promotion." September, 1991. NIH Publication No. 91-3216.

Winick, Myron, M.D. "The Role of Nutrition." *Menopause Management*, November/December, 1992; Vol. 1, No. 3, pp. 17–25.

Woolf, Anthony D. "Osteoporosis: Whose Problem Is It?" *Annals of Rheumatic Disease*, January, 1992; Vol. 51, No. 1, pp. 130–133.

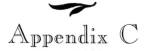

Appendix C

Papers Presented

Drinkwater, Barbara, Ph.D. "Physical Activity as A Key to Independence for the Older Woman." The North American Menopause Society 3rd Annual Meeting, September 17–20, 1992; Cleveland, Ohio.

Favus, Murray J., M.D. "Other Therapeutic Options in Osteoporosis." Program Syllabus for the meeting, Clinical Management of the Patient with Osteoporosis, September, 1992, National Osteoporosis Foundation.

Heaney, Robert, M.D. "Estrogen-Calcium Interactions at the Menopause." The North American Menopause Society 3rd Annual Meeting, September 17–20, 1992; Cleveland, Ohio.

Notelovitz, Morris, M.D., Ph.D. "Technology and Basis for Practice of Climacteric Medicine." The North American

Appendix C

Menopause Society 3rd Annual Meeting, September 17–20, 1992; Cleveland, Ohio.

Winick, Myron, M.D. "Nutrition, Menopause and After." The North American Menopause Society 3rd Annual Meeting, September 17–20, 1992; Cleveland, Ohio.

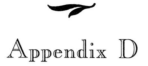

Appendix D

Self-Help Resources

Action on Smoking and Health (ASH)
2013 H Street NW
Washington, DC 20006

A Friend Indeed (a newsletter for women in the prime
of life)
P.O. Box 1710
Champlain, NY 12919-1710
           or
P.O. Box 515, Place du Parc Station
Montreal, Canada H2W 2P1

American Association of Retired Persons (AARP)
1909 K Street NW
Washington, DC 20049

Appendix D

American Cancer Society
1599 Clifton Road
Atlanta, GA 30329

American Dental Association
Department of Public Information and Education
211 East Chicago Avenue
Chicago, IL 60611

American Diabetes Association
National Service Center
1660 Duke Street
Alexandria, VA 22314
Call toll-free: 1-800-232-3472

American Dietetic Association
430 North Michigan Avenue
Chicago, IL 60611

Elderhostel
(Educational experiences for older adults based on
campuses throughout the country)
100 Boylston Street, Suite 200
Boston, MA 02116

Midlife Women's Network
(a newsletter)
5129 Logan Avenue S.
Minneapolis, MN 55419-1019

National Council on Aging (NCOA)
600 Maryland Avenue SW
West Wing 100
Washington, DC 20024

National Council on Alcoholism, Inc.
1151 K Street NW, Suite 320
Washington, DC 20005

National Institute on Aging (NIA)
Information Center
P.O. Box 8057
Gaithersburg, MD 20898

National Osteoporosis Foundation
1150 17th Street NW, Suite 500
Washington, DC 20036-4603

North American Menopause Society
c/o Department of OB/GYN
University Hospitals of Cleveland
2074 Abington Road
Cleveland, OH 44106

Osteoporosis Society of Canada
P.O. Box 280, Station Q
Toronto, Ontario M4T 2MI

Glossary

Bisphosphonates   Chemical compounds that impede resorption by inhibiting the action of osteoclasts, which are the bone-resorbing cells. There are a number of these compounds under investigation to see whether they successfully can serve as a treatment for osteoporosis.

Bone   The structural material of the body's skeleton that was formed from collagen, a soft protein, which has hardened by the addition of the mineral calcium phosphate.

Bone Mass   The actual amount of material contained in the bone. This mass increases quickly in adolescence, slowing down until about the age of thirty-five, reaching peak bone mass at about that time, and then declining. The amount of bone mass one has is an excellent predictor of fracture risk.

Glossary

Bone Remodeling A natural continuous process in which small amounts of bone break down and then are rebuilt by new bone tissue. This process occurs in two phases: the resorption phase during which old bone is broken down by the osteoclasts, leaving pitlike depressions; and the formation phase during which osteoblast cells deposit protein fibers and calcium to fill in those pits in the bone.

Calcium The mineral in the body which is the most abundant and is essential for building strong bones and for other important functions of your body, such as blood clotting.

Calcitonin A natural hormone secreted by special cells in the thyroid gland, it inhibits bone resorption. In patients with osteoporosis, synthetic salmon calcitonin treatment slows bone resorption.

Cortical Bone This is the outer shell of our bones, comprised of densely packed layers of tissue. The skeleton is made up of 80 percent cortical bone.

Dual-Photon Absorptiometry (DPA) One type of test that measures bone mass. It uses units of electromagnetic energy called photons at two levels (from a radionuclide source) to measure the total bone-mineral content, both cortical and trabecular, of the hip, the spine, and full body.

Dual-Energy X-ray Absorptiometry (DEXA)   A test that measures bone mass that uses photons (generated by an X-ray tube) at two energy levels. This test is faster and more precise in its measurements of the hip, spine, and full body and has less radiation exposure than Dual-Photon Absorptiometry.

Dowager's Hump   One of the most common visible signs of osteoporosis, this upper-back deformity is medically called dorsal kyphosis.

Estrogen   A hormone produced by the ovaries, estrogen influences bone mass by slowing or halting bone loss. It also helps retention of calcium by the kidney and improves absorption of dietary calcium by the intestine. When the natural estrogen is depleted due to menopause, estrogen replacement therapy (ERT) may be undertaken to restore it. Women with an intact uterus often take progestin with estrogen in therapy. This is referred to as HRT.

Osteoblast   A cell that makes and deposits new bone.

Osteoclast   A cell that reabsorbs and removes old bone.

Osteoporosis   A disease characterized by low bone mass in the skeleton, which leads to fragile bone and increased risk of fractures. There are two types of osteoporosis: Type I develops as a result of menopause and lack of estrogen; Type II occurs during the natural aging process in both men and women.

Parathyroid Hormone   This hormone is secreted by the parathyroid gland, which controls the level of calcium in the blood and kidneys by regulating the actions of the osteoblasts and osteoclasts. The parathyroid hormone and vitamin D work together in the body to maintain an appropriate level of calcium in the blood.

Photon   A unit of electromagnetic energy that is absorbed at a different rate by bone than by soft tissue.

Quantitative Computerized Tomography (QCT)   A technique by which radiographic X-ray beams measure trabecular bone density in the spine; the results are computer analyzed.

Radiographic Absorptiometry (RA)   A measurement of bone-mineral density from X-rays of the hand that undergo computer analysis.

Single Photon Absorptiometry (SPA)   A measurement of bone-mineral density using photons at a single energy level in the heels, forearm, and wrist.

Sodium Fluoride   A chemical compound undergoing investigation because of its ability to increase bone mass by stimulating osteoblast activity.

Trabecular Bone   The interior portion of the bone, trabecular bone has a porous spongelike structure.

Vertebrae   The thirty-three bones that compose the spinal column. Seven vertebrae are in the cervical spine in the neck; twelve vertebrae are in the thoracic spine in the chest; five vertebrae are in the lumbar spine in the lower back; five fused vertebrae are in the sacrum; and four fused vertebrae are in the coccyx.

Vitamin D   This is a nutrient that aids in calcium absorption from the intestine into the bloodstream. Too much vitamin D can be more dangerous than too little.

Index

Index

bones (*cont.*)
in men vs. women, 6, 32–33, 42,
    58–59, 91–92, 142
porous, 30, 31, 35, 36, 70, 152
rebuilding of, 29, 97, 107, 111,
    156, 176
stress on, 107–108
teeth vs., 61–62
breast cancer, 7, 55, 159–161
breast-feeding, 34, 65–66, 77–78, 101
breathing, difficulties with, 152

caffeine, 36, 57, 59, 79, 99, 100, 127,
    160
Calcimar, 168
calcitonin, 29, 104, 157, 165, 168,
    191
calcium, 85, 175, 177, 191
in bloodstream, 59, 71
bone strength and, 31, 38, 41, 73,
    77, 157
daily intake of, 60, 65, 102, 124,
    127–128, 159, 160, 162, 181
definition of, 125–127
dietary, 34, 35, 36, 47–48, 56, 63,
    77, 101–102, 128–129, 130,
    143–151, 166, 169, 176, 178,
    180; *see also* nutrition
estrogen and, 157–158, 166
and excessive protein, 98–99
fluoride and, 169–170
lactose intolerance and, 77, 137
measurement of, *see* bone-density
    tests
in men vs. women, 150
nighttime loss of, 132, 138
phosphorus and, 59, 60, 98, 99,
    140
soft drinks and, 59–61, 79, 99–100
taken with other foods vs. alone,
    138–139
toxic levels of, 60, 103, 136

vitamin D and, 69, 128, 139–140,
    167, 170
calcium carbonate, 131–132, 133
calcium citrate, 131–132
calcium-rich menu, sample, 143–151
calcium supplementation, 26, 28, 35,
    66, 77, 95, 96, 98, 104, 110,
    124–151, 166, 176, 184
best-absorbing, 133
determining need for, 130–131
digestive tract and, 139
ERT and, 157–158
fiber and, 134, 138
iron and, 134–136, 138
see also nutrition
calories, 77, 119, 175
Caltrate, 132
cancer, 7, 55, 167
ERT and, 45, 103–104, 159–161
Caucasian women, 34, 56, 78, 122,
    127
cereals, 133, 134
calcium-fortified, 101, 130
cesarean sections, 48
cheeses, 101, 137
childhood, bone-building in, 76–77,
    101, 102, 125
cigarette smoking, 36, 56, 63, 67, 89,
    90, 160, 175, 178
passive, 71–72
climbing, 182
clinical trials, women in, 5, 39–40,
    142
collagen, 31
computerized tomography (CAT
    scan), 85
coronary vascular disease (CVD),
    135
cortical bone, 31, 84, 85, 111
corticosteroids, 57, 73
cortisone, 63, 68, 71, 161
cyclosporine A, 73

Index

Index

Index

Index

About the Author

An award-winning medical writer and former vice president at Cleveland's prestigious Mt. Sinai Medical Center, Ruth S. Jacobowitz is author of *150 Most-Asked Questions About Menopause* and is the coauthor of *Managing Your Menopause*. Her lively, informative lectures on menopause have taken her all over the country, and she has been featured on such television programs as *Donahue*, the *CBS Morning Show*, *Jerry Springer*, *Company*, *Good Company*, *Northwest Afternoon*, *Morning Exchange*, and *People Are Talking* as well as in numerous major newspapers and magazines. She is a founding member of the North American Menopause Society and a former Midwest chair of the Association of American Colleges Group on Public Affairs. Mother of three married daughters and grandmother of four, she and her husband, Paul, live in Cleveland, Ohio.